Nursing in Nursing Homes

Other books of interest

The Care of Wounds: A Guide for Nurses
Carol Dealey
0–632–03864–0

Care of People With Diabetes: A Manual of Nursing Practice
Trisha Dunning
0–632–03876–4

Bolden & Takle's Practice Nurse Handbook
Third Edition
Gillian D. Hampson
0–632–03692–3

Understanding and Management of Nausea and Vomiting
Jan Hawthorn
0–632–03819–5

The Royal Marsden Hospital Manual of Standards of Care
Edited by Joanna M. Luthert and Lorraine Robinson
0–632–03386–X

The Royal Marsden Hospital Manual of Clinical Nursing Procedures
Edited by A. Phylip Pritchard and Jane Mallett
0–632–03387–8

Professional Discipline in Nursing, Midwifery and Health Visiting
Second Edition
R.H. Pyne
0–632–02975–7

Nursing in Nursing Homes

Linda Nazarko
BSc (Hons) Gerontology, RN

**Blackwell
Science**

© Linda Nazarko 1995

Blackwell Scientific Ltd
Editorial Offices:
Osney Mead, Oxford OX2 0EL
25 John Street, London WC1N 2BL
23 Ainslie Place, Edinburgh EH3 6AJ
238 Main Street, Cambridge,
   Massachusetts 02142, USA
54 University Street, Carlton,
   Victoria 3053, Australia

Other Editorial Offices:
Arnette Blackwell SA
1, rue de Lille, 75007 Paris
France

Blackwell Wissenschafts-Verlag GmbH
Kurfürstendamm 57
10707 Berlin, Germany

Blackwell MZV
Feldgasse 13, A-1238 Wien
Austria

First published 1995

Set by DP Photosetting, Aylesbury, Bucks
Printed and bound in Great Britain by
Hartnolls Ltd, Bodmin, Cornwall

DISTRIBUTORS

Marston Book Services Ltd
PO Box 87
Oxford OX2 0DT
(*Orders:* Tel: 01865 791155
        Fax: 01865 791927
        Telex: 837515)

North America
   Blackwell Science, Inc.
   238 Main Street
   Cambridge, MA 02142
   (*Orders:* Tel: 800 215-1000
           617 876-7000
           Fax: 617 492-5263)

Australia
   Blackwell Science Pty Ltd
   54 University Street
   Carlton, Victoria 3053
   (*Orders:* Tel: 03 347-5552)

A catalogue record for this book is available
from the British Library

ISBN 0–632–03987–6

Library of Congress
Cataloging in Publication Data
is available

Dedication

To my husband without his support, guidance and advice this book would not exist. Thanks Ed.

Contents

Preface

Ten years ago there were few nursing homes. Older people were looked after in NHS hospitals. NHS care included acute, rehabilitation, ongoing and palliative care. There were few nursing homes and people who required long-term care were nursed in geriatric hospitals or units in acute hospitals. The nursing homes which did exist were a world away from the nursing homes of today. Now nursing homes provide 168 000 places nationally for older people, while the NHS has only an estimated 35 000 long-stay beds[1].

The number of very elderly people (those over the age of 85) has grown. At the beginning of the century there were only 50 000 people over the age of 85 and by the end of the century there will be about 1.2 million[2]. It is estimated that a further 70 000 places will be required by the end of the decade and that the majority of those places will be in nursing homes[3]. While ageing is not an indicator of an individual's abilities, people are more likely to suffer from health problems as they age. Older people take longer to recover after illness and their recovery is often dependent on the skills of elderly care nurses. Nurses who work in partnership with older people to identify and meet the older person's needs can ensure that individuals retain and regain skills.

NHS changes have emphasized increased 'patient throughput' and the criteria by which hospitals are often judged is how many people have been treated within budgetary constraints. Older people spend less time in hospital following major illness or accident than previously. Staff are under enormous pressure to discharge patients early so that more can be treated[4]. Older people are now discharged to nursing homes more acutely ill than ever before. Some older people do not even enter hospital. At times when hospital beds are at a premium, such as in the depths of winter, older people who are perceived to have nursing needs are admitted to nursing homes directly from hospital accident and emergency departments. Older people living in nursing homes who require hospital treatment, perhaps for a fractured femur following a fall, are discharged within a few days of surgery[5]. Others who require investigations such as gastroscopy, or surgery such as cataract removal and implantation of intra-ocular lens, are dealt with on a day-case basis.

The implementation of the Community Care Act has accelerated these changes. Most nursing home patients require a greater degree of skilled nursing care than ever before.

There are now over 70 000 nurses working in nursing homes[6]. They come from a variety of backgrounds. Some are experienced elderly care nurses who came to work in nursing homes when local NHS long-stay facilities were closed. Some are nurses who have returned to nursing after a break at home to raise a family and others are newly qualified nurses who have come to work in nursing homes immediately after qualification.

There are important differences between nursing homes and NHS elderly care units, both in the way they function and the nursing skills required. These are illustrated in Table P.1.

Table P.1 Differences between nursing homes and NHS elderly care units.

Nursing homes	NHS elderly care units
Nurse led	Consultant geriatrician in charge
GP 'on call'	Doctor on site
Nurse determines admission	Nurses have no control over admission
Senior nurse 'on call'	Senior nurse 'on site'
Infrequent interaction with colleagues working in other nursing homes	Frequent interaction with colleagues on other wards
More likely to feel isolated	Less likely to feel isolated
May lack policies and procedures. Any which exist will be drawn up by nurses working in the nursing home	Existing policies and procedures may refer to the entire hospital rather than be specific to the elderly care unit
Supervision of ancillary staff rests with nurses	Nurses are not responsible for supervising ancillary staff
Greater responsibility for obtaining, recording and auditing medication	Hospital pharmacists are employed
Vital role in referring patients to other professionals	Other professionals 'on site' to deal with referrals

The nurse who begins work in a nursing home may feel overwhelmed by the variety of roles required. Nothing in nurses' training or NHS experience prepares them for an important role within a nurse-led unit. Nursing in nursing homes is exciting, challenging and satisfying. This book aims to help guide the nurse through the uncharted waters of nursing home nursing, to work in accordance with the UKCC Code of Conduct, to satisfy legal requirements and to deliver the best possible nursing care.

This book covers the following topics: Chapter 1 deals with the legal framework; Chapter 2 explains assessing and admitting patients; Chapter 3 deals with challenging behaviours; Chapter 4 covers the ordering, custody and safekeeping of medication. Chapters 5, 6 and 8 are concerned with infection control and wound care, and continence promotion is discussed in Chapter 7. Chapter 9 deals with safety and risk management, Chapter 10 discusses nutrition and Chapter 11 is about obtaining services. Areas new to nursing homes – rehabilitation and respite care are discussed in Chapters 12 and 13. Chapter 14 is concerned with palliative care and death with dignity, and the final chapter deals with the future in nursing homes.

Elderly care is an area where nursing makes a vitally important contribution to an individual's quality of life. That contribution is of critical importance in nursing homes. This book aims to provide nurses with the information and advice they require to enable them to nurse well involving the patient in all aspects of care. It aims to encourage and advise the nurse in caring for individuals in a holistic, humane and sensitive way. It stresses the importance of avoiding isolating different aspects of nursing as such factors as the individual's psychology, mobility, medication, and diet are all equally important. It encourages the nurse to work with the older person, their family and friends, together with other professionals, to provide the best possible care. Nursing homes are full of people with a lifetime of experience – working with them is not only rewarding, it can also be great fun. Enjoy your work!

Unfortunately it has not been possible to cover every aspect of nursing home nursing in this book. I would be pleased to receive readers' comments and suggestions, which can be sent via the publisher.

All names used within the text are pseudonyms.

References

(1) Laing, W. (1994) *Care of Elderly People; market survey*. Laing & Buisson.
(2) OPCS (1991) Mortality Statistics. Serial tables 1845–1985. Office of Population Censuses and Surveys, London.
(3) Laing, W. (1994) *Care of Elderly People; market survey*. Laing & Buisson.
(4) News: Survey shows big drop in NHS bed availability. *Nursing Times* (1993), 89, 49, 8.
(5) GLACHC (1994) *London Hospitals Discharging their Responsibility?* Greater London Association of Community Health Councils, London.
(6) Hansard (1994), Written Answers 14 January 1994, Column 316 (Relates to period 1992–93).

Linda Nazarko
January 1995

Acknowledgements

The author would like to thank Smith & Nephew for permission to use the frequency volume chart reproduced in Chapter 7 (Fig. 7.1).

Figs 8.1 and 8.2 are taken from C. Dealey (1994) *The Care of Wounds*, Blackwell Science Ltd, Oxford.

Chapter 1
The Legal Framework

Introduction

Nurses working in nursing homes must satisfy the requirements of the relevant legislation. For nursing homes in England, Wales and Northern Ireland the relevant legislation is the Registered Homes Act 1984[1]. Nursing Homes in Scotland are governed by the Nursing Homes Act 1939. Nurses also have professional responsibilities under the United Kingdom Central Council (UKCC). Nursing homes are subject to inspection by law. These inspections are carried out by registration and inspection teams on behalf of the local health authority. This chapter discusses the role and responsibilities of registered nurses working in nursing homes. It also explores the role and responsibilities of registration officers in relation to the relevant legislation and the UKCC code of conduct.

Legal requirements

At present UK nursing homes are subject to rules and conditions laid down in the Registered Homes Act 1984. Scottish legislation is the Nursing Homes Act 1939. The Registered Homes Act lays down conditions of registration, inspection and record keeping within homes. These conditions concern not only matron/managers but all registered nurses working in nursing homes.

Each home is required to be registered with the local health authority. The health authority issue a registration certificate which gives details of the category of registration and the number of patients who can be cared for in the home. This must be displayed in a prominent place in the home and failure to do so is an offence under the Act. A fee is charged by the health authority for initial registration. An annual registration fee is then charged to the home on the anniversary of the original registration. The current fee for registration is £22 per bed. It is claimed that this fee fails to cover the cost of running inspection teams and there have been calls to increase the annual charge to £50 per bed.

1

This would bring registration fees for nursing homes in line with the registration fees for residential homes[2]. Some registration authorities also charge a fee for posting information and circulars to homes; typical charges are £20–£30 per year. There is no provision under the Act to enable registration authorities to charge this.

The Act requires homes to be inspected at least twice every year. In practice this usually entails one annual visit when the home is given prior notice of inspection. At this visit all relevant documentation is normally examined. The second visit is normally an *ad hoc* visit and staff are not notified of the visit. The aim of this visit is to gain an insight into the running of the home. Some inspection teams are also incorporating a night visit into the inspection schedule so that visits give an indication of care throughout the day and night. Inspection and registration officers have a legal right to enter any nursing home on production of identification. They may ask to see records or ask the nurse in charge for information relating to records or day to day care within the home. According to the Act only a medical practitioner employed by either the Health Authority or the crown is entitled to view medical records.

Person in charge

The person in charge of the home is required to be a registered nurse or a registered medical practitioner. In practice the vast majority of people in charge are nurses. The person in charge is traditionally referred to as the matron. This title has been criticized by some who view it as dated and sexist. Nursing home patients, relatives and fellow professionals appear to understand and appreciate a traditional title which they understand. In some homes the person in charge is referred to as the manager – but patients and relatives often enquire if the manager is a qualified nurse as the title manager can be used by many people in a variety of occupations. In other homes the title director of nursing services is used – but this can appear pretentious especially in small homes and many patients do not understand its meaning.

The title matron will be used throughout this chapter to denote the person in charge. The matron is required to give written notice (wherever possible) to the inspectorate if away from work for more than four weeks. One month's notice should be given of planned absences. In an emergency situation the matron is required to give notice of absence no more than one week after the absence commenced. On return the matron should give notice of return within a week of resuming duty. Details of the proposed length of absence and arrangements made to manage the home in the matron's absence will be required. These should include the name, address and qualifications of the person managing the home in matron's absence.

Record keeping

The matron is required by law to keep certain records. A register should be kept of all patients admitted; this should include details of name, address, GP, date of birth, and date of discharge or death. Such records are legally required to be kept for one year. It is good practice to retain such records for seven years in case they should be required for legal reasons.

The home should keep a separate record of all surgical operations. In nursing homes these would normally be dental extractions and occasional minor operations carried out under local anaesthetic such as removal of ingrowing toe nails, warts or small lipomas. The Act states that these records should be retained for one year but it is good practice to retain them for seven years.

An adequate daily statement of the patient's health and condition must be kept. Most homes use printed care plans and progress notes which are held in plastic sleeves in folders. The progress notes satisfy conditions relating to daily records. The UKCC recently commented that completing these written records on a daily basis regardless of the patient's condition 'wasted nurses' time'[3]. Completing these records reminds nurses that they should be vigilant at all times to the possibility of any change in a patient's condition. Details of investigations and treatment are also required. Using care plans and progress reports and noting investigations such as urinalysis, weight and blood tests in these records satisfies the provisions of the Act.

A record of staff employed at the home, which includes name, date of birth, dates of employment and qualifications, must be kept at the home. Normally an indexed book or loose leafed folder is considered satisfactory.

Details of fire practices, fire alarm tests, fire procedures and action taken to remedy defects must be kept. All staff working within the home should have training on fire drill every six months[4].

Details of maintenance to equipment must be kept. This includes routine maintenance of equipment such as lifts, cookers, dryers and hoists. This equipment may be serviced by the manufacturers as part of a service contract. In this case details of work carried out at each visit are given by the contractor (usually a loose leafed sheet). These should be retained for a minimum of one year.

Homes are required under the Act to give written notice of death to the health authority within 24 hours of a death occurring within the home. Most registration officers supply pre-printed forms which are completed by the nurse in charge of the shift when the death occurred. These forms normally ask the cause of death. If a post mortem is required the inspection officer should be notified in writing (retaining a copy for the home's files) of the death. The cause of death can be supplied and the form completed when this is known.

The Act assigns duties and responsibilities to the 'person registered'. This is normally the proprietor or in the case of a large company it may be the managing director. In some homes the person registered is also the matron; this tends to occur mainly when the matron is also the proprietor, but it can occur in other cases. The registered person has responsibilities under the act to ensure the provision of:

- adequate staff including ancillary staff
- adequate space including day room space
- adequate furniture, beds, screens to ensure privacy
- adequate medical and nursing equipment and facilities
- adequate lighting, maintenance, cleanliness and decor
- adequate fire precautions and staff training
- adequate kitchen equipment, food and laundry facilities
- adequate arrangements for disposal of clinical waste
- adequate arrangements for patients to receive medical and dental services
- adequate arrangements for the recording, safekeeping, handling and disposal of drugs
- adequate arrangements for prevention of infection
- adequate arrangements for occupation and recreation
- adequate privacy
- adequate precautions against the risk of accident.

In practice the company or proprietor may delegate these functions to the matron. In these circumstances the matron is provided with budgets and facilities to enable these criteria to be met.

The United Kingdom Central Council (UKCC) Code of Conduct

All nurses will be familiar with the UKCC Code of Conduct which is issued to all registered nurses, midwives and health visitors[5]. The code clearly states '. . . you are responsible for your own practice . . .'.

The code comprises 16 points which outline the nurse's duties and responsibilities.

Nurses in nursing homes, like nurses in other areas of practice, may be placed in situations where they are asked or directed to take action which contravenes the code. A patient's doctor may request that a wound is cleaned with Eusol. The research evidence which indicates that the use of Eusol on wounds is damaging is incontrovertible; details are given in Chapter 6. The UKCC Code of Conduct, clauses 1 and 2, state:

(1) Always act in such a manner as to promote and safeguard the interests and wellbeing of patients and clients.

(2) Ensure that no action or omissions on your part, or within your sphere of responsibility, is detrimental to the interests, condition or safety of patients and clients.

In the situation of using Eusol, as mentioned above, if the nurse were to comply with the doctor's request she would be in breach of the code. The nurse can discuss the research evidence with the doctor and inform him of the wide range of alternative treatments now available which render the use of substances such as Eusol obsolete.

Catherine King had been employed in a senior position in a nursing home for three years. The home, part of a small nursing home group, was sold. The new proprietor, who was not a nurse, asked Catherine for the nursing records as she wished to be fully aware of each patient's medical and nursing needs. The UKCC Code of Conduct clearly states in clause 10:

> 'Protect all confidential information concerning patients and clients obtained in the course of professional practice and make disclosures only with consent, where required by law or where you can justify disclosure in the public interest.'

Catherine informed the proprietor of this and explained that she could not allow the proprietor access to the records for this reason. Catherine assured her that the skilled professional nursing staff were the people qualified to make decisions on clinical matters.

Sue Daniels was visited by a newly appointed nursing home inspector at 3 AM one morning for a routine night visit which was part of the local inspectorate's policy. The inspector checked records, medication and staffing as normal. She then stated that she wished (discreetly and causing minimal disturbance to patients) to check each patient's bottom to ensure that pressure sores were not present. The UKCC Code of Conduct, clause 7, states that the nurse should 'recognize and respect the uniqueness and dignity of each patient and client...'. Sue felt that the registration officer's request contravened clauses 1, 2 and 7 of the code of conduct. She explained that she was unable to allow this and requested that the inspector returned in the morning to discuss this with matron if she still wished to inspect the patients' bottoms. The inspector discussed this with the senior inspecting officer the next day and apologized as such action would have been utterly inappropriate and totally unprofessional.

The Code states in clause 6 that nurses should:

'work in a collaborative and co-operative manner with healthcare professionals and others involved in providing care, and recognize and respect their particular contributions within the care team.'

Some nurses feel that this section of the Code prevents them from challenging other professionals when they witness behaviour which is not of a professional standard. Some feel that if a more senior person asks them to do something they must comply. *The nurse's prime responsibility is not towards employers, doctors or senior nurses it is to ensure that patient care is of the highest possible standard.*

Patients and their families trust and respect professional trained nurses. Nurses care for the most vulnerable and disabled people of their generation in nursing homes and have a duty to act in the patient's best interest at all times. It can be difficult for nurses to refuse to accede to the wishes of people more powerful and influential than themselves. The nurse should explain politely and reasonably the ethical dilemmas which such requests raise and how they conflict with the code of conduct. In many cases the individual concerned will have been unaware of the implications of such requests and will reconsider their actions. The nurse can, if she is unsure of the ethical and professional implications of a request, defer any action until she has consulted matron or her professional organization.

The role of registration and inspection officers

Registration officers have a legal duty to inspect nursing homes. The legislation requires them to carry out two visits each year. One of these, the annual visit, is arranged with the matron and the registered person. The second visit is normally on an *ad hoc* basis. Increasingly registration officers are including a night visit in this schedule. The purpose of inspection is to ensure that the care given is satisfactory, that the matron is competent, that the home is adequately maintained, that the home is complying with legislation and that the person registered is competent. The nursing home inspector has a legal right to enter the premises at any time but must provide proof of identity. If the nursing home inspector has concerns about the quality of care visits may be more frequent.

Registration officers are responsible for assessing the 'fitness' of the matron under the legislation. In a situation where the person registered sought to appoint a newly qualified nurse or a nurse without post registration experience in elderly care, the nursing home inspectorate would object. Health authorities have the power to cancel the home's registration if they have evidence that the matron is 'not fit', though the inspectorate will use this power only as a last resort. The Royal College of Nursing has published guidance on the role and qualifications of nursing home matrons, which is available free to RCN members[6].

Registration officers also have a role to act as a nursing resource. This includes working to educate and inform nursing home staff.

Nursing home inspectors are appointed by health authorities. Some health authorities consider inspection of nursing homes to be of prime importance. They employ sufficient numbers of nursing home inspectors to enable them to carry out their duties, and inspectors are paid salaries which reflect the importance of such posts. Unfortunately some health authorities do not consider the inspection of nursing homes a high priority. This is reflected in the number of inspectors appointed, the salaries offered and the qualifications and experience required for the post.

Nurses come to the inspectorate from a variety of backgrounds. Some have significant experience and post registration qualifications in elderly care, whilst others do not. There are no nationally agreed guidelines specifying the experience and qualifications required for the post of a nursing home inspector. Currently the only training available to nursing home inspectors is at the National Association of Health Authorities and Trusts (NAHAT). The training available to inspectors varies from 1 to 5 days. A recent report recommended 'all those undertaking registration and inspection to receive comprehensive training'[2].

Nursing home inspections

Recent research indicates that 24% of inspections are undertaken by a single inspector, 33% by two inspectors and 43% by a team involving four or more people[6]. The inspection team can consist of one or more inspection officers, an environmental health officer, a fire officer, a district pharmacist, a health and safety officer, and a secretary to the inspectorate. The time an inspection takes can vary from two hours to twelve hours.

Advocates of inspection teams state that this is an efficient method of inspection. Most nurses who have experience of being inspected by a team of four or more people find this extremely disruptive and that it can be detrimental to patient care. The environmental officer may spend an hour or more with the chef and catering assistant. The pharmacist may spend two or more hours conducting a pharmacy audit with a trained nurse. The fire officer, accompanied by a trained nurse, will inspect fire procedures and question staff about their knowledge of fire drills. The health and safety officer, accompanied by a member of trained staff, will check health and safety procedures, discuss staff knowledge training and procedures relating to legislation, check hoists and lifts and ask to see evidence of maintenance.

Matron and the registered person will be accompanying the inspection officer who is checking relevant documentation, inspecting the building and chatting to patients and staff. Matron will be constantly interrupted by the other inspectors who all wish to ask relevant questions. This method of inspection can be intimidating, disruptive and fails to give the inspectors a true picture of life within the home. Nurses who feel that the relationship between the inspection team and the home is a coercive one and not one based on mutual professional respect may hesitate to consult the inspectors when they require advice.

Inspection by one or two inspection officers indicates a more professional relationship where nurses can work together with the common aim of ensuring the highest possible standards of care for the patients. The environmental health officer can visit the home twice yearly, as required, on a different occasion and can spend time inspecting the home and talking with staff. The fire officer can combine inspection visits with fire drills and can answer staff questions and queries and work with staff to ensure patient safety. If the home is subject to visits from a large team and the nurse feels the disruption entailed is detrimental to patient care, the inspection team should be informed of this in writing. It may be possible to restrict the team visit to the annual notified inspection. Adequate arrangements can then be made to ensure that appropriate numbers of staff are on duty to continue with patient care whilst the inspection is in progress. This normally involves having twice the usual number of nursing staff on duty for the duration of the inspection and a few hours afterwards.

Registration officers either publish their own guidance about the standards required in nursing homes or refer to a document produced by NAHAT[7]. Less than half of inspectors have developed a quality audit tool to enable them to audit standards within the home[6]. Following the inspection the inspectors issue a written report, which they are required to send to the registered person. The matron or registered person can then reply to any concerns or can challenge any aspect of the report with which they disagree. In recent years increasing numbers of inspectors have been sending a copy direct to the matron. This practice has been frowned on by some proprietors but it seems fair and reasonable that the person in charge is fully aware of all details of an inspection. The matron is then in a position to act on any concerns relating to nursing care.

It is good practice for the matron to show inspection reports to all staff and to discuss any issues in detail with senior staff. If the report praises aspects of the home's care then showing it to staff boosts morale. Any areas which require further work can be discussed and explored by staff who can work together to improve them.

The Act fails to define standards and practice precisely and much is left to the interpretation individual inspectors place on the legislation.

This can cause problems on occasion; for example an inspector might favour a particular nursing model such as the Orem model, whilst matron and staff prefer to use an alternative model such as the Roper, Logan and Tierney model. The inspector can suggest that the Orem model is more appropriate in certain circumstances but cannot tell staff which model they should use.

Staffing levels

The nursing home inspector issues a 'staffing notice'. This details the *minimum* levels of nursing staff required on each shift within the home and will give details of how many registered nurses and how many care assistants are required on morning, afternoon and night shifts. Nursing home inspectors in some areas use a staffing matrix to determine staffing levels. Other factors such as the layout of the home, patient dependency and facilities available are taken into consideration when staffing levels are determined. The ratio of qualified staff to care assistants has risen in recent years as the dependency levels of patients has increased. The registered person or the person in charge has the right to appeal against staffing levels which appear unreasonable.

Some nurses occasionally find that the nursing home proprietor wishes to appeal against staffing notices and reduce the ratio of qualified to unqualified staff. The nurse should be aware of sections 11, 12 and 13 of the UKCC Code of Conduct. If the nurse feels dilution of skill mix would place patients at risk she should explain this to the registered person. Often nursing home proprietors who do not come from a professional nursing or medical background are unaware of the value and cost effectiveness of skilled professional nurses. The RCN produce a booklet (free to members) which nurses in such situations will find valuable[8].

It must be emphasized that the staffing levels specified by the inspectorate are minimum staffing levels. In some situations, when workload is particularly heavy, perhaps because a number of patients are ill or require a member of the nursing staff to escort them to out-patients appointments, additional staff will be required.

Dealing with complaints

The nursing home should have a philosophy which enables older people to make real choices about how they lead their lives in a nursing home. Regular patients meetings, the use of primary nursing and staff who are open, approachable and welcome suggestions usually mean that any minor problems can be quickly resolved. In this atmosphere there are few complaints. The home should however have a policy for dealing with complaints. Complaints should be dealt with as quickly as possible and in a sensitive and sympathetic manner. Most complaints are dealt with in the home in such an atmosphere. If the home is unable to resolve complaints they may be referred to the inspection officers.

Some relatives and friends do not discuss complaints directly with staff at the home but complain directly to the inspector. The inspector will visit the home to discover if there are any matters for concern. It can be very upsetting for nursing staff who were unaware of any problems to discover from an inspector that a formal complaint has been made. Skilled nursing home inspectors will deal with complaints in a sensitive way and will investigate any allegations. A written report will be issued and the matron (or nurse concerned) can respond in writing. Often complaints are simply a matter of staff and patients or relatives failing to communicate properly and not understanding each other's role. Nursing home inspectors can help nursing staff and patients or relatives rebuild lines of communication in such cases and resolve any problems within the home.

Conclusion

The aim of legislation, the UKCC Code of Conduct and the nursing home inspectorate's work is the same as that of the nurse: to ensure that older people living in nursing homes receive the highest possible standards of care. Nurses must be aware of the requirements of legislation and the UKCC Code of Conduct if they are to fulfil their requirements. It is important that the nurse forms a professional working relationship with fellow nurses working as inspection officers and that all professional nurses work together towards the common aim of ensuring quality care is delivered.

References

(1) *The Registered Homes Act 1984.* HMSO, London.
(2) *An Inspector Calls?* The Regulation of Private Nursing Homes and Hospitals. (1994) Royal College of Nursing, London. This is free to RCN members; contact your local regional office (address in RCN diary issued free to members).
(3) Concern over new deregulation bill (1994) News story in Nursing Standard, **9**, (7) 8.
(4) Draft guide to fire regulations in existing residential care premises. 1985 Statutory Instrument SI 1984 no. 1578 Regulation 12 (1) e (1).
(5) *UKCC code of professional conduct* (1992) (3rd edn). UKCC, London.
(6) *The Role of the Nursing Home Matron* (1995) Royal College of Nursing, London.
(7) *The Handbook on the Registration and Inspection of Nursing Homes* (1984). National Association of Health Authorities and Trusts (NAHAT), Birmingham.
(8) *The Skill and Value of Nurses* (1993) Royal College of Nursing, London.

Chapter 2
Assessing and Admitting Patients

Introduction

Older people seldom seek nursing home care. They prefer, naturally, to remain at home. Older people are usually persuaded to consider moving to a nursing home when it is no longer possible to provide the level of care they require in another environment.

There are different categories of nursing homes which provide care to differing groups of people. There are homes for individuals with learning difficulties. These are staffed by nurses with Registered Nurse Mental Handicap (RNMH) qualifications and usually care for people below retirement age. Homes registered for Elderly Mentally Infirm (EMI) provide care for older adults with mental infirmity and are staffed by Registered Mental Nurses (RMN). The majority of nursing homes are registered to care for Elderly Infirm and are staffed by Registered General Nurses (RGN). Some larger homes are run as two units; one for Elderly Infirm individuals and one for Elderly Mentally Infirm. Each unit must have a minimum of one appropriately qualified registered nurse on each shift. Minimum staffing levels are set by the registration and inspection team in consultation with the nursing home proprietor and matron/manager.

Homes are registered to provide care to women over the age of 60 and men over the age of 65 years. Most people who live in nursing homes are in their 80s and 90s. The average nursing home patient is almost 84 years old[1].

Older people are often persuaded to consider nursing home care because of the worsening of chronic physical or mental problems. An older person with worsening arthritis who is no longer able to cope with the activities of daily living, even with full community support, might be persuaded to consider nursing home care.

Until recently older people admitted from home were less frail than individuals admitted from hospital. The introduction of the Community Care Act (CCA) in 1993 has changed this. Individuals admitted from home frequently require high levels of skilled nursing care.

Many older people who have been cared for in Social Services homes by untrained staff are referred to nursing homes when they require high levels of nursing care. Individuals are also referred from residential care. Most older people are referred to nursing homes from hospitals. In many cases an individual has been living independently at home until illness strikes, perhaps a severe cerebro-vascular accident. Individuals who fail to recover sufficiently to return home are advised to seek nursing home care. The thought of never returning home and of going into a home can be a great shock to an older person and their family. Usually older people requiring nursing home care are not well enough to contact nursing homes, visit them and choose a suitable home themselves. Relatives are usually asked to do this on an older person's behalf.

How Social Services Departments assess the need for nursing home care

The Community Care Act was introduced in April 1993. This act gave local Social Services Departments (SSDs) the 'lead responsibility' in assessing which older people required long term care. SSDs were allocated budgets to purchase care. Prior to the CCA individuals requiring nursing home care could apply for benefit from the Department of Social Security. There were no overall limits to the DSS budgets. The budgets allocated to SSDs are limited so criteria were introduced to decide who required nursing home care. This normally involves an assessment with a points system. An individual must score a certain number of points to be referred for nursing home care.

Each individual SSD has worked out their own system. Assessments are carried out either by nursing staff or care managers. Many care managers have been employed recently; some have social work or nursing qualifications but some are unqualified. If an individual is assessed as requiring nursing home care this is discussed with the individual and family members. Relatives are normally given a list of homes and asked to find a suitable one. If an older person has no family or close friends then care managers seek a suitable home.

The role of trained nurses in assessing and admitting patients

Many relatives are understandably shocked and upset when asked to find a nursing home. Most are unfamiliar with the different types of homes and have little idea of the care their relative requires. Some newly appointed care managers are unsure of the differences in homes registration. Nursing homes are nurse-led units. They are run by a qualified nurse who is responsible for assessing the care an individual requires and working with trained nursing staff, ancillary staff and other professionals to ensure that care is delivered. The matron/manager is normally responsible for all aspects of running the home, including admitting individuals to the home.

Matrons have a responsibility under the Registered Homes Acts[2] to provide appropriate care to individuals admitted to the home. They also have a responsibility under the United Kingdom Central Council (UKCC) Code of Conduct in this respect. Matrons can only admit individuals if they are satisfied that care needs can be met; for example, if an older person has a tracheostomy and requires frequent suctioning to maintain the airway then a suction machine and a back-up system must be available. If an individual was admitted and these facilities were not available, the nurse could be found guilty of misconduct in the event of a case being referred to the UKCC.

It is essential that matron or a senior member of her trained staff visits any individual requiring nursing home care and carries out a full nursing assessment before agreeing to admit that individual. Assessment and obtaining details of an individual's medical, nursing and social history enable the nurse to have a clear picture of the care an individual requires. This assessment should include an assessment of the individual's mental state and any behaviour which could affect the wellbeing of the individual or other residents of the home. Individuals who tend to become confused and wander off, perhaps trying to return home, would be at risk if the nursing home is situated on a busy main road.

The assessment should include how much help the individual requires with the activities of daily living. Problems such as deteriorating eyesight or deafness often only become apparent when an older person is assessed by medical or nursing staff. If matron is assessing an older person in hospital and is informed that communication is difficult because of a hearing problem, matron can suggest that an audiology referral is organized before discharge. The older person can then return, as an outpatient, for further help. Assessment should include dietary needs, details of past medical history and current medication.

Individuals may have been receiving nursing care, perhaps from a district nurse for a leg ulcer or from a continence adviser for a continence problem. A nursing history and details of treatment and progress will enable nursing home staff to offer continuity of care. An example of a nursing assessment form is shown in Fig. 2.1.

An assessment visit allows the older person to meet a member of staff and to find out as much as possible about the home. Nurse and patient have an opportunity to chat about how the home is run and discuss the aims of care. The assessing nurse should make every effort to be present when an individual whom she has assessed is admitted. The older person will naturally feel apprehensive about coming to stay in a nursing home and a friendly greeting from a familiar face can be helpful and reassuring. Placing a simple bunch of flowers and a few treasured

NURSING ADMISSION SHEET

Name:	Room Permanent/Temporary
Address:	D.O.B. Age Date/Time admitted:
Tel No:	Accompanied by:
Marital Status:	
Religion:	Type of Admission: Emergency Waiting List
Next of Kin:	Reason for Admission:
Relationship:	
Address:	Confirmed Diagnosis:
Tel No:	
Contact in Emergency:	Patient aware of reason for admission:
G.P.	Urinalysis Weight:
Address:	Past Medical History *(serious illnesses & hospitalisation)*
Tel No:	
Lives alone: Yes/No	
Property: *if any valuables are stored, state what and where*	
Discharge/Transfer	
When:	
Where to:	Allergies:
Transport:	
Reason:	Investigations and Date:
TTAS:	
Relatives informed:	
General Appearance:	Vision:
Mobility—help needed	Elimination:
Walking Dressing	Urinary:
Bathing Eating	
Comments:	Bowel:
Mental State:	Nutritional State:
Comments:	Dietary Preferences:
	Special Diet:
Skin State:	Sleep:
Broken Areas:	Usual Pattern
Norton Score:	Sedation
Oral Inspection:	Pain—Description:
Dentures Full/Partial	
Hearing:	Leisure Activities, Interests:
Uses Aid	
	History taken by:
	From:

Fig. 2.1 Patient assessment sheet.

possessions in the room before the individual arrives can make the room welcoming.

Funding care

There are 4500 nursing homes in the UK. Some homes are run by charities and these usually only consider certain categories of older people for admission. An older person may have to be a resident of a certain area or have worked in a specific occupation. The remainder of homes are run as businesses. All homes have set fees; most charges are based on the type of room occupied rather than the care required. Single rooms are in most cases more expensive than shared rooms. Fees vary according to the standards of accommodation provided and the home's location. Single room fees vary from £300 to £700 per week and shared rooms from £290–£500 per week.

Financial assessment

Nursing home care is means tested. Individuals with capital, property or assets of more than £8000 must pay their own fees. If an older person owns a house then they must sell the house to pay for care. If the older person has a husband, wife (or in some cases a relative) living in the house then the value of the house is excluded from the financial assessment. Older people who have all their capital tied up in their home have nursing home fees met by SSDs until the house in sold. Some SSDs then reclaim the fees paid from the older person's assets, whilst other SSDs do not.

Financial assessment takes into account an older person's income including occupational pensions. Social Services Departments are responsible for purchasing care on behalf of older people who have assets of less than £8000. Social Services Departments also take over responsibility for payment of nursing home fees when individuals who have entered care after April 1993 have used their own capital. Details of benefits available to older people who entered a nursing home before April 1993 are given in the section in this chapter on DSS funding and preserved rights. The responsibility for purchasing care rests with the area the older person lives in and not the area they may wish to move to. An older person who wishes to move from Ipswich, for example, to be near family in Glasgow remains the responsibility of Ipswich who must fund care.

Negotiating with Social Services Departments

In April 1993 SSDs were, for the first time, allocated budgets to purchase nursing home care for older people living in their area requiring such care. Budgets were allocated from government based on the numbers of older people living in each area. These budgets did not take into account the numbers of older people able to self fund. In more affluent areas SSDs found themselves funding only a small proportion of nursing home placements; in other areas SSDs have funded almost all nursing home placements. When SSDs were informed of their budget allocations they drew up budgets and worked out how much they could afford to pay for nursing home care. Most SSDs then contacted nursing homes in their area and asked them if they wished to contract with the SSD. Homes wishing to do so were expected to have certain facilities and had to meet certain criteria. These vary from area to area and are reviewed at intervals of 1 to 3 years.

In some areas SSDs demand higher standards of accommodation and apply more stringent standards than registration departments. Many stipulate that individuals are not cared for in multi-occupied rooms. Double rooms are acceptable but many SSDs prefer to contract with homes who have a ratio of 80% single rooms to 20% double rooms. Many SSDs demand evidence that the home is financially sound. They are increasingly asking for details of staff training programmes and are wary of contracting with homes that have a high turnover of staff.

These checks are to ensure that SSDs are purchasing quality care from reputable homes. Homes are then asked how much they would charge for care. Individual homes or nursing home groups then negotiate with SSDs and both parties agree the price of care within the home. These negotiations have resulted in SSDs paying very different prices for care in homes in the same area. Many SSDs are, it appears, prepared to pay a premium for quality care and peace of mind.

These negotiated prices are known as base prices; in many areas they are much higher than the rates paid by the Department of Social Security (DSS) and have been calculated to take account of the higher levels of care now required. Social Services Departments are prepared to pay a premium when purchasing care for older people requiring extremely high levels of care. Some SSDs, perhaps fearful that their budgets would run out, set fee levels at the same rate as DSS payments. In areas where homes contract with a number of SSDs those offering DSS levels find it difficult to obtain places for older people from their area. Social services fees range from £295 to £385 per week outside London and from £350 to £450 within the London area. Homes in some areas, especially large cities, negotiate care with a number of SSDs within travelling distance. Homes who have negotiated with SSDs are then placed on the SSD's list of approved homes. This list gives basic details of the home's location, facilities, the name of the matron/ manager and the negotiated fee levels. This list is given to older people or their relatives who use it to select a suitable home.

Individual contracts

Older people requiring nursing home care are normally allocated a care manager. Care managers help older people and their families to select homes and work with nursing home staff to arrange admission. When a home has been selected and admission confirmed the care manager carries out a financial assessment. This assessment details the cost of care and who is responsible for paying it.

Individuals who are funded by SSDs have part of the fees met by payments from DSS benefit and part from Social Services. Individuals who have income from other sources, for example an occupational pension, have this taken into account. All older people in nursing homes are allowed to retain a 'personal allowance' (currently £13.40 per week) for personal needs. The care manager then draws up a contract for each individual placement. This contract imposes certain conditions on the nursing home, normally referred to as 'the provider', on the SSD, normally referred to as 'the purchaser', and on the older person or a family member, who may sign on their behalf. A plan of care is normally drawn up at this stage and forms part of the contract.

How fees are paid

Individuals admitted under the Community Care Act (CCA) who are entitled to SSD help have a finance form included in their contracts. This details the home's fees, income support payable, SSD payments and any element of fees which relatives may have agreed to pay. Relatives are not obliged to pay towards fees but in some cases where SSD and income support payments do not meet the full cost, relatives may choose to contribute to fees. This might happen when SSD and income support benefits cover the cost of a sharing room but relatives wish to pay for a single room. An example of a financial contract is given here:

Mrs Jones' savings = less than £3000.
Homes fees = £375 (weekly costs of care in a London nursing home).
Income from Social Security income support = £110.30.
Social services payment = £264.70.
Personal allowance = £13.40 weekly, is paid in addition to the above amounts and intended to enable individuals to buy personal items and clothing.

The contract will give details of how SSD payments will be made. Normally invoices are sent to SSDs every four weeks and payment for the SSD component is made directly to the home either by cheque or credit transfer.

The income support component of payment must be applied for by the older person or the family, who complete a form SB1 which is sent by the local DSS office. Income support can now be paid either by order book or directly into the older person's bank account. The home invoices the older person directly for this proportion of the fees. In many cases older people living in homes are unable to cope with their financial affairs and these are managed by a friend or relative.

Appointee status

Older people who are unable to manage their own financial affairs can appoint someone else to collect benefits and manage their affairs. Normally older people in this situation are visited by a DSS visiting officer who meets the older person and the person willing to become an appointee. Appointees are usually close friends or relatives and they must sign a form promising to use benefit for the purposes issued: paying fees and providing for the older person's needs.

Nursing staff as appointees

Some older people do not have any close relatives or friends able to act as appointees. On other occasions the appointee can become ill and no longer able to carry on. In these circumstances a senior member of the home's staff, usually the matron, is asked to become appointee. The DSS will approve this 'in exceptional circumstances'. Appointeeship involves a lot of work for nursing staff. Benefit must be collected, the proportion paid to the home must be paid and the personal allowance collected for the individual. Appointeeship involves keeping scrupulous records of all benefit and these may be checked by DSS or registration officers.

Many nurses have taken on the onerous duties of appointeeship only to discover that the older person has many relatives. Nurses should agree to become appointees only if they are absolutely sure there is no friend or relative available.

Admission to hospital

Older people who have been admitted to hospital from a nursing home either under the CCA or under preserved rights suffer no loss of benefit provided their stay in hospital does not exceed six weeks. A hospital stay of more than six weeks is rare as hospitals tend to discharge older people living in nursing homes earlier than they would those living at home, because skilled nursing care is available in homes.

Care reviews

The purpose of a care review is to visit the older person in the nursing home and review the care required. Care managers discuss the placement with the individual and family and with nursing staff. They check that the individual has settled in, is content, that care needs are being met and that the placement is appropriate. Long and short term aims are identified and care needs discussed and documented. If the placement is proving successful and appropriate a further care review is carried out six months later.

Caring for extremely dependent older people

It is not uncommon for nursing homes to care for individuals who a few years ago would have been cared for in hospital. Older people are frequently admitted to homes with pressure sores or at extremely high risk of developing sores. Such individuals require specialist equipment such as low air loss beds.

Nurses who are caring for older people who require high levels of care have a duty to provide the care required. Dependency scales can be used to demonstrate to care managers the levels of care required. The ENAZ dependency score is based on an individual's ability to carry out activities of daily living. The lower the score the greater the level of dependency. Dependency scores can be used to monitor an individual's progress, to demonstrate the level of care required and to determine staffing levels. Social Services Departments are usually prepared to a pay a premium when purchasing care for extremely dependent older people. They are usually willing to pay for the hire of, or arrange loan of, specialist equipment from local hospitals.

Hospitals were allocated funds under the Community Care Act and can purchase care directly from nursing homes for individuals with high care needs. Normally such placements are negotiated individually and charges reflect the levels of care required. The charge for caring for an individual in a vegetative state requiring gastrostomy feeding, passive movements and intensive nursing care varies from £800–£1000 per week. A copy of the ENAZ dependency scale is shown in Fig. 2.2.

Placement of older people with mental health needs

Individuals living in nursing homes are usually in their 80s and 90s. The incidence of Alzheimer's disease and Alzheimer's type dementia (ATD) rises with age. Alzheimer's disease is a physical disease which causes a progressive decline in the ability to remember, to learn, to think and to reason. Nursing homes registered to care for Elderly Mentally Infirm individuals employ RMN trained staff who are specially trained to care

Score patients on skills in activities of daily living (ADL) listed below. The higher the score the lower the level of dependency. Tick the appropriate boxes.

		Scores			
		0	1	2	3
Feeding:		☐	☐	☐	☐
Independent	= 2				
Needs help	= 1				
Dependent	= 0				
Dressing:		☐	☐	☐	☐
Independent	= 2				
Needs help	= 1				
Dependent	= 0				
Mobility:		☐	☐	☐	☐
Independent walking	= 3				
Minimal help	= 2				
Independent in wheel chair	= 1				
Immobile	= 0				
Chair/bed transfer:		☐	☐	☐	☐
Independent	= 3				
Minimal help	= 2				
Moderate help	= 1				
Totally dependent	= 0				
Mental state:		☐	☐	☐	☐
Orientated	= 2				
Mildly confused	= 1				
Confused at all times	= 0				
Safety:		☐	☐	☐	☐
Minimal risk	= 2				
Moderate risk	= 1				
High risk	= 0				
Bladder control:		☐	☐	☐	☐
Fully continent	= 2				
Occasionally incontinent	= 1				
Incontinent/catheter	= 0				
Bowel control:		☐	☐	☐	☐
Fully continent	= 2				
Occasional incontinence/					
or enemas required	= 1				
Faecally incontinent	= 0				
Grooming:		☐	☐	☐	☐
Independent	= 1				
Dependent	= 0				
Bathing:		☐	☐	☐	☐
Independent	= 1				
Dependent	= 0				

Fig. 2.2 ENAZ dependency scale.

for older people suffering from dementia. Many Social Services Departments pay a premium to EMI registered nursing homes. This premium, typically £20 to £30 per week reflects the high levels of care individuals with advanced dementia require. EMI nursing home beds are in short supply in many areas and tend to be reserved for older people with advanced dementia.

The onset of dementia is gradual and it can be difficult for medical and nursing staff working in community, hospital or nursing home settings to recognize it. Physical illness, medication and transfer to a new environment can all cause older people to become disorientated. It would be impossible to accommodate in an EMI home every older person who is becoming forgetful or has a period of mild confusion. Individuals who have been living in a nursing home for some time can develop dementia. If an older person has come to regard the nursing home as 'home' and nursing staff can provide the required care medical staff and registration officers normally agree that moving the older person to an EMI registered home would be inhumane.

Some older people who develop dementia or mental health problems cannot be cared for effectively within nonspecialist nursing homes. The individual's behaviour may be dangerous to themselves or others. In an acute situation the individual's GP can usually arrange for an emergency appointment with a psychogeriatrician and hospital admission can be arranged if necessary. In less urgent cases an appointment can be made with a psychogeriatrician and if necessary arrangements made to transfer the individual to an EMI registered home as soon as possible. Relatives can be extremely distressed by such transfers. Great sensitivity is required in such situations. The reasons for the move to another home should be explained. The nurse can give details of nearby EMI homes and suggest the relative visits and chooses a suitable home. The older person's care manager should be informed of any change in care needs and of any plans to transfer to another home.

Attendance allowance

Attendance allowance is an allowance which individuals can claim to help them meet the costs of care. It is not means tested. Older people living in nursing homes, who are receiving DSS benefit or whose care is funded by Social Services, will have benefit adjusted to take account of attendance allowance if they receive it. Older people who are funding their own care normally claim this benefit. Claim forms can be obtained from the local DSS office or the post office. Individuals are not normally considered for this benefit unless disability has persisted for more than six months. Terminally ill individuals are exempt from this ruling. There are two levels of attendance allowance: the higher rate allowance is for individuals who require assistance throughout the day and night and the lower rate is for individuals who only require assistance during the day. The higher rate is currently £45.70 and the lower rate is £30.55.

DSS funding and 'preserved rights'

Some older people who enter homes and fund their own care eventually exhaust their capital. They often ask nursing staff to advise them what benefits they are entitled to when their capital reaches £8000, the level at which they are eligible for help. Older people admitted prior to April 1993 should apply to their local Department of Social Security who will send a form (SB1) which must be completed to claim benefit. These individuals have been allocated DSS preserved right status and are able to continue to claim DSS income support. Individuals keep preserved rights status even if they move to different homes.

There are special arrangements for individuals who have been funding their own care before 29 April 1985 and individuals in this situation should contact their local DSS office for further details. They must emphasize that they have been funding their own care prior to 29 April 1985. Before the CCA was introduced there were fears that SSDs would offer fee levels lower than the current income support levels; preserved rights status was a measure to protect older people in nursing home care.

Current benefit levels under preserved rights are £296 outside London and £325 in London. However SSDs have at least matched, and in many areas exceeded, DSS fee levels. DSS fee levels fail to cover the costs of care in some homes and although many nursing home proprietors have continued to accept DSS fee levels from existing residents they are unable to admit individuals with preserved rights. Social Services Departments are not able to offer help with fees in such circumstances. Many individuals with preserved rights find themselves unable to transfer from residential to nursing home care or from one home to another unless they can find additional funds.

Sources of additional funding

Many organizations have benevolent funds which will consider helping older people with their fees. Many occupations such as the police force have benevolent funds. Individuals who were members of a trade union should contact the union as many have benevolent funds. There are hundreds of charities and benevolent funds who may be able to help. Older people and their families often lack the time and resources to track down possible sources of funding. A number of organizations will help relatives to find additional funding.

The Elderly Accommodation Council (EAC) is a charity which aims to help older people locate and fund suitable accommodation. They produce a questionnaire which individuals are asked to complete. Details from the questionnaire are then used to check through over 800 charities, and individuals are advised which charities should be approached. Every case is dealt with individually.

> Elderly Accommodation Council,
> 46A Chiswick High Road,
> London W4 1SZ
> Telephone 0181 742 1182.

Age Concern provides a number of fact sheets which give advice and information on sources of additional funding and many other topics. The charity also has an information line and will answer individual queries.

> Age Concern (England)
> Astral House
> 1268 London Road
> London SW16 4ER
> Telephone 0181 679 8000.

Counsel & Care provide information and run an advice line.

> Counsel & Care
> Twyman House
> 16 Bonny Street
> London NW1 9PG
> Telephone 0171 485 1556.

Charity Search provides free advice for elderly people and links them with charities which may be able to help with funding.

> Charity Search
> 25 Portview Road
> Avonmouth
> Bristol BS11 9LD
> Telephone 0272 824060.

Useful addresses and telephone numbers

(Use this to enter local information relevant to your work)

Local care managers

Social Services finance departments

Department of Social Security

References

(1) Baldwin, S., Corden, A. *et al.* (1990) *A Survey of Nursing Homes and Hospices.* Centre for Health Economics and Social Policy Research Unit, University of York.
(2) The Registered Homes Act 1984 covers England, Wales and Northern Ireland. In Scotland the Registered Homes Act (1939) applies.

Chapter 3
Challenging Behaviours

Introduction

Individuals whose need for care arises primarily because of mental health needs should be cared for in nursing homes registered to care for Elderly Mentally Infirm (EMI). These individuals should be cared for by registered nurses with a qualification in mental health nursing (Registered Mental Nurse). Nurses working in non EMI nursing homes often care for individuals who suffer from confusion and who display behaviours such as wandering, screaming, shouting and aggression. These behaviours may arise as a result of physical or mental illness. Some older people may have been admitted to the home for physical care and may develop dementia.

The Alzheimer's Disease Society estimates that 25% of people over the age of 85 develop a dementing illness. This can pose an ethical dilemma for nurses: is it ethical to transfer a long term resident because they develop dementia and the home is not registered to provide such care? It is more humane to continue to care for the older person in familiar surroundings, but how will this affect the other patients? Will they become upset and worried by unpredictable and challenging behaviour? The aim of this chapter is to give the nurse an insight into the causes of confusion and the reasons older people develop challenging behaviours. This will enable the nurse to plan care which minimizes or eliminates challenging behaviour.

The causes of confusion

Confusion is not an inevitable result of extreme old age. There is always a reason for confusion. When an older person becomes confused the nurse's first reaction should be to ask why.

There are many physical causes of confusion. Often the first sign of an older person developing an infection is confusion. Temperature, pulse and respirations may be normal but the normally lucid older person has become confused. If an older person suddenly becomes confused the nurse should check temperature, pulse, respirations and blood pressure. She should ask the older person if they feel unwell and should observe the individual carefully. Have they developed a cough which may indicate a chest infection. Are they passing urine more frequently? Have they become incontinent? Does the urine smell? If a urinary tract infection is suspected the nurse should test urine and if nitrite or protein is present should follow the infection control procedure for the home. Is the older person very thirsty? If glucose is present in the urine the GP should be contacted as untreated diabetes is a major cause of confusion in older people. Does the older person appear pale, tired and listless? Anaemia can cause confusion. Electrolyte imbalance and uraemia can also cause acute confusional states in older people.

Head injury can lead to subdural haematoma (bleeding into the dura between the brain and the skull). A slow dural bleed is more likely to cause confusion than a rapid bleed. If head injury is suspected the doctor should be contacted immediately. Surgical evacuation of subdural haematoma by a neurosurgeon restores function if the individual is referred in time.

Medication can often cause confusion. Night sedation can cause individuals to become extremely confused and some antidepressants can cause older people to develop delusions.

Medication given to control the symptoms of Parkinson's disease can cause acute confusional states. Steroid therapy which is reduced too quickly can cause the individual to hallucinate. The nurse should check if medications have been altered recently or if the individual is taking prescribed medication which could be leading to confusion.

Older people who slowly become confused are often assumed to be suffering from dementia. It is important to exclude physical causes of confusion before assuming that an individual is suffering from an irreversible terminal disease. Older people who suffer from hypothyroidism may appear to be suffering from dementia as the lack of thyroid hormone slows mental function. A simple thyroid function test enables the GP to check if hypothyroidism is responsible for mental deterioration. Thyroid deficiency is easily treated with thyroxine, and mental function is restored. Individuals who suffer from Parkinson's disease may be diagnosed as suffering from dementia if they are not carefully examined. If Parkinson's disease is treated older people can often enjoy a long period of normal life.

Daisy Jenkins, a retired confectioner and baker, slipped on an icy pavement and fractured her femur. This was pinned and plated in hospital but Daisy was unable to return home as she was unable to care for herself. Her primary nurse noted that Daisy's face was an expressionless mask and she appeared rigid and still. Daisy constantly rubbed her index finger and thumb together. On admission Daisy's sister explained that she was not surprised that Daisy had fallen as for some months she had been shuffling along and not picking up her feet.

The primary nurse suggested to the GP that Daisy might be suffering from Parkinson's disease. This was found to be the case and the disease responded to treatment. She was discharged home after a period of rehabilitation and visits the nursing home every Christmas and Easter with Christmas and simnel cakes which she bakes and decorates herself.

Bereavement and grief can cause people of all ages to lose interest in life and to become muddled. Some older people are admitted to nursing homes because a carer who provided physical care has died. Overwhelming grief, sense of loss and the admission to a nursing home can cause an older person to become confused.

Depression can cause agitation, sleep disturbances, self neglect and disinterest in surroundings.

Dementia can cause confusion. Dementia is a global term used to describe a group of diseases which affect the brain. Dementia affects memory first. It can take some time for memory loss to become apparent and it is estimated that most people are not diagnosed as suffering from dementia until two years after the onset of the disease. Eventually all aspects of thinking and reasoning are affected. The commonest causes of dementia in older people are Alzheimer's disease and multi-infarct dementia. Alzheimer's disease is often diagnosed by doctors but it is only possible to confirm diagnosis by examining brain tissue under a microscope. If the individual has not had a brain biopsy then the diagnosis of Alzheimer's is unconfirmed.

There have been a number of reports in the press in recent years suggesting that if an individual suffers from Alzheimer's then other family members may develop the disease when they become older. Many families are worried that they may also develop dementia in old age. The nurse may have to reassure families that research into genetic factors is in its early stages and that families of individuals who develop dementia in old age are at no greater risk of developing the disease than anyone else. It is only the families of people who develop early onset dementia in their 40s and 50s who have an increased risk of developing dementia.

Multi-infarct dementia is more common in men, is of sudden onset and is associated with arterial disease, caused by small clots which lead to the death of areas of brain tissue. It can be diagnosed by a brain scan which shows small areas of brain death caused by brain infarctions. Treatment of arterial disease and hypertension can prevent or reduce the frequency of further brain infarctions.

Lewy body disease is thought to be a type of Alzheimer's but deterioration is more rapid[1]. Parkinson's disease can lead to dementia in approximately 30% of sufferers. This dementia normally develops in the later stages of the disease. Pick's disease, frontal dementia and Huntingdon's chorea are other causes of dementia, but onset is usually before the age of 65.

Caring for people suffering from confusion

Confusion caused by physical problems will resolve following treatment. People suffering from intense overwhelming grief and depression will normally recover following treatment and counselling. Nurses can help by taking time listen to them when they wish to express their feelings.

A team approach is of the utmost importance in caring for long standing residents who develop dementia and are to remain in the home. Even in the early stages of dementia individuals benefit from a consistent approach to care. *The most important aspect of caring for older people who develop dementia is to avoid premature disablement.* Nursing staff may treat an individual with dementing illness like a child and this can hasten the individual along the continuum to disability. The individual should continue to be treated with respect and called by his or her preferred title. The goal of skilled nursing care should be *to enable not to disable.* If an individual finds it difficult to dress the nurse should ask why. Sleeves may be too tight and buttons too small; dresses which fasten at the front rather than the back and clothing which is easy to put on may enable the individual to continue dressing themself.

An older person suffering from dementia may appear to take a long time to eat. Staff, fearing that the meal will get cold or that senior staff will be unhappy if meals are not finished and dishes cleared by a specific time, may feed the individual. The nurse should adopt a problem solving approach. Why is the individual taking so long to eat? Are they chatting with other residents and taking their time? This is perfectly reasonable behaviour and the member of staff who rushes to feed the individual is the one behaving abnormally. All staff should be aware that the resident's right to enjoy a relaxing meal takes precedence over any routine chores. The nursing home is the older person's home, not an institution run for the convenience of the staff. We have all lingered over restaurant meals in good company but the waiters, however badly they wish to go home, do not feed us. Dining rooms in nursing homes can be busy and full of bustle, and this can be distracting to some individuals suffering from dementia. Promoting a quiet calm atmosphere and keeping distractions to a minimum may be all that is required.

Other residents, domestic staff, the individual's family and the families of other residents can all undermine care by 'helping' the confused individual with activities of daily living. Domestic staff may feed an individual, the older person's roommate may dress them or comb their hair, visitors who would never dream of helping lucid residents may treat a confused individual like a child. The nurse needs to ensure that all staff are aware of the aims of care, and should observe patients, visitors and families carefully, intervening if they are undermining nursing care.

Communicating with individuals suffering from confusion

Communication is vital if the nurse is to understand and meet the needs of an individual suffering from dementia. Nurses are busy people and often bustle around giving individuals little time to communicate their needs. It is important that nurses slow their pace and spend time finding out what the needs of the individual are. Dementia is a continuum and the skills required to communicate effectively with individuals who are at different stages of that continuum are very different.

Ensuring that there are not too many distractions is helpful. Some individuals may find watching the domestics clean up far more interesting than talking to the nurse. The nurse should use short sentences and wait for a reply. Only one idea should be expressed in each sentence. Simple plain language should be used. Abstract concepts should be avoided. Check that what you say has been understood. Check that you understand what the individual has said. The nurse should be aware of any other disabilities such as hearing loss or dysphasia, and should use strategies to enable the individual to communicate. Further details are given in Chapters 11 and 12.

Touch is a powerful way of communicating and the nurse should use touch to emphasize and improve communication. Listening is even more important than speaking. The nurse should listen to what the individual is saying and learn to interpret what the individual has said. Nurses should check that they have understood the meaning of words by saying 'Do you mean . . .?' The nurse must work with all staff who come in contact with the confused individual and teach them how to communicate and recognize a confused individual's needs. This ensures that the whole team are working together in harmony to meet the individual's needs. Problem behaviours are less likely to occur when staff are able to communicate with and meet an individual's physical and emotional needs.

Wandering

The older person who appears to wander aimlessly around the home can disturb other residents. Staff attempting to cope with wandering behaviour can feel anxious, worn out and inadequate. They may fear that the individual will have an accident and they will be blamed. Residents' relatives may complain about individuals who wander, asking 'Can't the doctor give them something?'. Sedation though can worsen the situation rather than improve it. Often the individual continues to wander but is at greater risk of injury because of the effects of sedation.

The reasons individuals wander

Wandering is *not* an aimless activity. The older person has a reason for wandering and the aim of skilled nursing care is to discover the reason. When the nurse has identified this it is possible to work out a strategy to modify behaviour. All older people do not wander for the same reasons[2]. Wandering is not related to the degree of confusion or the stage of dementia an individual has reached[3].

People who wander may have difficulty in communicating their needs. Wandering may be an attempt to satisfy those needs. The nurse must use a range of skills to discover the reasons for wandering. Closely observing the individual, talking to the individual, staff, family and friends and investigating any possible causes can often uncover the reason the individual is wandering.

Observation of gestures and movements and an awareness of the individual's medical history may suggest that the individual is suffering from pain. The causes should be investigated and treated by the individual's doctor.

The individual may wish to use the toilet but may be unable to find it. Opening all the doors in a corridor may be a quest to find the toilet. Toilets with large clear signs and staff directing the individual to the toilet can eliminate wandering. The individual may be constipated, uncomfortable and unable to communicate this to staff. Instead he may visit the toilet frequently and remain there for some time.

The individual may be hungry and looking for food. The diet in the home may be sufficient for inactive older people but insufficient to meet the needs of an active older person. Are second helpings of food available? Are snacks offered? Has the individual a tin of biscuits or a bowl of fruit? The individual may be thirsty; are drinks left in bedrooms and lounge areas so that residents can help themselves? The individual may be looking for possessions such as a book or handbag which have been left behind in the bedroom. The individual may be bored stiff and has decided to go for a walk. The lounge may noisy and full of bustle and the individual has decided to escape from the noise and find somewhere quiet.

Wandering at night

Wandering can be a particular problem at night. Again the nurse should find out the reasons for wandering. The individual may feel lost and lonely in the dark. They may always have slept alone and find it difficult to sleep in a room with another person. They may have shared a room with a spouse for many years and feel alone and cut off in a single room. The older person might need only five or six hours sleep but is encouraged to go to bed at 7PM; by 1AM they are awake and bored. The individual may be hungry. What time is the evening meal served? The individual may not know what time it is. Is there a clock in the room? Does it show the correct time or has someone forgotten to wind it or change the batteries? Can the individual see the clock? Is the home on a busy main road? Does the roar of traffic wake them?

Managing wandering behaviour

Wandering behaviour can be managed and in many cases eliminated if the nurse discovers the reasons for the behaviour. As there is no one single reason for wandering there can be no single solution. The nurse who finds the reason can ensure that the older person's needs are met and the need to wander is reduced or eliminated. The individual who longs for a brisk walk may find that a daily walk with a staff member to the shops not only removes the need to wander but is also a pleasant experience. The individual who is suffering from pain and discomfort will become less restless when pain is treated. The individual who keeps wandering into the kitchen looking for food need not do this if they are provided with food and snacks to prevent hunger.

Shouting, screaming and singing

The individual who constantly calls out, screams or sings the same song over and over again can upset other residents. Staff often feel unable to cope with such behaviour; and the individual who shouts or screams may be moved from home to home. Sedation may be prescribed by doctors in a vain attempt to control behaviour. There are no easy solutions to manage these behaviours. The goal of skilled nursing care is to identify the reasons for them and adopt a problem solving approach.

The reasons why individuals scream, shout or sing

There are many reasons why individuals behave in this way. They may not realise they are shouting if they are not wearing their hearing aid because staff did not help to put in, or if the hearing aid is turned off or the batteries need replacing. Individuals who are dependent on glasses to see, or hearing aids to hear, or dentures to eat and who do not have these aids may become confused and disorientated as a result of sensory deprivation. Imagine how terrifying the home must appear to someone who cannot see or hear properly. The individual may be bored if none of the staff bother to talk to them and relatives seldom visit. A loud scream is an effective way of gaining attention.

The individual may be unable to communicate needs and can only call out 'help, help, help' in the hope that some one will understand and offer to meet their needs. They may be in pain, hungry, tired, thirsty, lonely. The lounge area may be busy and noisy, the television may be too loud. They may long to escape to the quiet of their bedroom but be unable to express these needs. They can only call 'nurse, nurse, nurse'.

The individual may call out continually for someone, a spouse or child perhaps. A knowledge of the older person's life can help the nurse to make sense of this behaviour.

> Mrs Eileen Barnes was frail but lucid when she was assessed for admission to a nursing home. She had left her home, entered hospital and been transferred to three different wards before her transfer to the home. On admission she was extremely confused and called out for 'Timmy'. Mrs Barnes was widowed, with no children or close family. Her primary nurse discovered that Timmy was her pet budgie and was being looked after by friends. The home had a policy which enabled older people to bring small pets with them on admission. Timmy joined Mrs Barnes in the home, her needs were met and the shouting stopped.

Nurses though cannot always meet needs so easily; a widow will never be able to see her husband again. Sometimes, though, the nurse can help by talking to the individual concerned:

'You must miss your husband John very much . . .'

'Yes, tomorrow is our wedding anniversary.'

The nurse, by acknowledging the individual's feelings and enabling the older person to express these feelings, created an atmosphere in which the woman could speak about her husband without having to shout to gain attention.

Managing challenging behaviours

Skilled sensitive professional nurses who discover the reasons why an individual is shouting, screaming or singing can adopt a problem solving approach and work with other members of the team to meet the individual's needs. Remembering that the individual who is shouting is a human being who may be feeling lost, lonely and afraid and is not a management problem, will enable the nurse to respond sensitively and meet the individual's needs to the best of her ability.

Aggression

Confused older people may hit out at staff or other patients. Staff behaviour may appear threatening to an older person who has difficulty in working out what the nurse's intentions are. The nurse who looms menacingly over the older person, invading their personal space, may only be placing a cup of tea on the older person's table. The nurse who removes bedclothes and disturbs the sleeping older person may wish to change a wet bed. The nurse who begins to undress an older person may wish to wash the individual. The older person may not realise this, perhaps because the nurse spoke too quickly or did not check that the individual understood and consented. In such situations the older person can lash out, pushing the nurse away, knocking over or throwing the tea, or punching the nurse who is attempting to remove clothing.

Nursing staff who explain and obtain the individual's consent before touching them find this lessens the likelihood of aggressive behaviour. If an older person has lashed out an incident form should be completed. Senior nursing staff should discuss possible reasons for the aggressive behaviour. Do staff lack skills and experience? Are staff inadequately trained? Are staff too busy and responding to work pressures by rushing an individual? Are staff ignoring the individual and only meeting physical needs? Does the individual feel angry and frustrated? Is movement painful?

It is often possible to eliminate aggressive behaviour if the reasons for its occurrence are uncovered and action taken to meet needs. In some cases, though, the older person can be aggressive towards other extremely vulnerable older people living in the home, who have done nothing to provoke such behaviour. Staff may also be subjected to unprovoked attacks. Older people and staff have the right to feel safe and secure within the home. The nurse must balance the needs of the older person who is displaying aggressive behaviour with the needs of others living and working in the home. The individual who is aggressive may require care from nursing staff with mental health qualifications and expertise.

Conclusion

There are many causes of confusion, and it is vitally important that the cause is identified. Physical illness should be treated and individuals who are suffering from depression or grief should be offered appropriate treatment and counselling. Confusion of sudden or gradual onset should never be dismissed as a result of age or diagnosed as dementia until all other possible causes have been investigated.

The prime aim of skilled nursing care should be to enable older people with dementia to retain existing skills for as long as possible and to avoid nursing practice which prematurely disables people. The nurse must develop a range of skills to enable her to identify the reasons why confused people behave in ways which we find difficult to understand. Identifying the reasons for behaviour will enable the nurse to meet the individual's needs, enhance the quality of care and in many cases eliminate or greatly reduce the incidence of challenging behaviour. There are no easy solutions.

The nurse must also recognize that not all problems can be solved in a nursing home staffed by general trained staff. Staff may be unable to manage behaviour. An individual's behaviour may be seriously affecting the quality of life of other older people living in the home. In these circumstances it is not appropriate to continue to offer care within the home. The individual's needs are primarily needs related to mental health. These needs should be met in a home registered for the Elderly Mentally Infirm, which is staffed by nurses with mental health qualifications and expertise.

Further reading

Harvey, M. (1990) *Who's confused?* Prepar Publications, Birmingham.

Stokes, G. (1988) *Wandering.* Winslow Press, Bicester.

Allan, K.M. (Ed) (1994) *Wandering.* Dementia Services Development Centre, Stirling University.

Stokes, G. (1988) *Screaming and Shouting.* Winslow Press, Bicester.

Alzheimer's Disease Society (1984) *Caring for the person with dementia.* Alzheimer's Disease Society, London.

References

(1) Cox, S.M. & McLennan, J.M. (1994) *A Guide to Early Onset Dementia.* Dementia Services Centre, Stirling University.

(2) Synder, L.H. et al: (1978) Wandering. *The Gerontologist.* 18, 272–80.

(3) Fopma-Loy, J. (1988) Wandering: causes, consequences and care. *Journal of Psychosocial Nursing,* 26, 8–18.

Chapter 4
Medication

Introduction

The Registered Homes Act contains one line on the ordering, administration and safe custody of drugs within nursing homes. It simply states that the person registered 'must make adequate arrangements for the recording, safe-keeping and disposal of drugs'.

Nurses working in nursing homes are responsible for ordering from the pharmacy, recording drugs supplied to the home, drugs which patients bring from home or hospital, and drugs returned to the pharmacy. They are responsible for the storage of medication and for monitoring usage and investigating discrepancies. This involves carrying out drug audits. They must ensure that all medication charts have been correctly written up and signed by local GPs. Nurses must either draw up or ensure that any policies relating to errors in drug administration are fair and just and protect both patient and staff.

Nurses who have moved to nursing homes from hospital or community practice have never been asked to carry out such duties before and nursing training does not prepare them for such duties. There is no national guidance on the role of the trained nurse in relation to medication and few articles have appeared in nursing journals. Few health authorities produce information on this subject. A recent report by the United Kingdom Central Council (UKCC) was critical of nurses' abilities to carry out their duties in relation to storage, administration and record keeping of medication[1]. This chapter aims to make nurses aware of good practice and to give practical help and advice in implementing good practice in their work area.

Choosing a pharmacist

Nurses who have been appointed to work in a new home will be approached by a number of retail pharmacists who are anxious to supply the home with a pharmacy service. Older people living in nursing homes receive medical care from GPs who prescribe medication by writing a prescription on a form FP10. Normally prescriptions are left with the home, who obtain the medication from a retail pharmacist.

Retail pharmacists are paid for each prescription item they dispense and nursing home business is extremely lucrative, so they compete with each other to supply nursing homes. Nurses are often unaware of this and arrange that the first pharmacist to approach them, or the nearest pharmacist, can supply the home. It is advisable for nurses to ask pharmacists what services they will supply before appointing. It is important that an out of hours service is available so that nurses can obtain emergency prescriptions 24 hours a day, 365 days a year, if required. This service should be available as standard and not given as a favour or grudgingly. A delivery service should be provided for regular and emergency items.

It is important to enquire if the pharmacist has a computerized system. Pharmacists with computer systems, or another method, can provide monthly or four weekly printouts of patient prescriptions, which can be used when auditing medication. They will also be able to supply records of an older person's usage of a particular medication going back months, if required for auditing purposes. Pharmacists should be willing to take part in drug audits and assist and advise nurses in implementing good practice.

Medication in nursing homes is prescribed to individuals. Enquire how the pharmacist proposes to deliver a monthly supply of medication. The pharmacist who delivers it jumbled up in a couple of cardboard boxes is wasting your time and does not deserve your business. Choose the pharmacist who will deliver every individual's medication in an individually labelled bag. This will save nursing time when checking medication received and will make it easy to store medication and find it in the stock cupboard when it is required.

If you find a number of pharmacists who can meet your requirements ask them which nursing homes they currently supply. The staff of another home will normally be pleased to tell you the pharmacist's good and bad points. A little time taken choosing a pharmacist will save so much time and trouble that it really is worth choosing your pharmacist with care. There is no reason why nurses should feel compelled to choose the nearest pharmacist, if a better service is available from a pharmacist some distance away and delivery arrangements are satisfactory.

Getting the best from an existing pharmacist

Many nurses inherit a pharmacist when they go to work in a home. A good pharmacist plays an important role in ensuring that a first class pharmacy service is delivered to a home. Sadly there are some pharmacists who do little more than dispense medication. Some nurses are expected to collect and deliver prescriptions and medication to their homes and are expected to use emergency pharmacists for out of hours services. Nurses who find themselves in such situations should meet with the pharmacist and negotiate a service such as that outlined in the section on choosing a pharmacist. Most pharmacists who are aware of nurses' needs and expectations will be eager to change and tailor their service to the home's requirements as they would not wish to risk losing the business.

Ordering medication

Medication is ordered on an individual basis for individuals in nursing homes. Stock medication cannot be ordered and stock bottles cannot be kept. If ten individuals are prescribed digoxin 62.5 mcg then ten individual prescriptions must be issued. Each prescription issued by a GP must have the individual's name and address on it. No more than seven items can be ordered on one prescription form (FP10). Prescription items are normally ordered every 28 or 30 days for all individuals in a home. Items such as a course of antibiotics are ordered when prescribed and for a set number of days.

When a GP has supplied a prescription the nurse completes the back of it on the individual's behalf. She indicates, by ticking a box, that the individual is over retirement age (and thus entitled to free prescriptions) and stamps and signs the prescription. Details of all prescriptions ordered should be entered in a bound book kept specially for this purpose. The book should have details of date ordered, name of patient, drug ordered, dose, and amount of medication ordered. The book should also have details of date of delivery and space for two nurses to sign when the medication is received. This book provides a record of all medication received into the home. Individuals who enter the home from hospital or the community should have any medication which they bring in with them entered in this book. Failure to do this can cause problems when auditing medication.

Controlled drugs

It is good practice to record any controlled drugs ordered in red and to write the amount ordered in words and figures.

Non-prescription medicines

In some areas the home and the district pharmacist agree a written list of non-prescription medicines which nursing staff may give without a prescription. These items normally include paracetamol and cough medicines. The agreement stipulates the length of time these may be given, usually between two to four days.

This practice is fraught with danger for both patient and nurse. It almost certainly contravenes UKCC guidance on standards of administration of medicine. The majority of older people in the home will already be taking prescribed medication. There may be a danger of drug interactions. An older person prescribed a drug such as thioridazine who is given a cough linctus containing codeine could become very drowsy. If they were to fall, fracture a femur or even die, the nurse could be held responsible.

There is also the danger that medication will mask symptoms which require medical investigation and treatment. An individual with a history of hypertension who develops a headache may be suffering from severe hypertension, or acute glaucoma which, if untreated, can cause blindness.

Nurse prescribing will become more widespread in the future. Nurses will be required to undertake additional training before being permitted to prescribe. Nurses who dispense unprescribed medication under locally agreed protocols should consider the UKCC Code of Conduct Clause 4:

'... and decline any duties or responsibilities unless able to perform them in a safe and skilled manner.'

Storing medication

As all medication is prescribed and dispensed on an individual basis, storage of medication can be difficult. Homes should have a drugs trolley (or trolleys) with individual drawers for each individual. All medication in current use for the individual should be stored in the drawer. Additional bottles and packs of medication can be stored in bags with the individual's name on the bag, in a locked cupboard, preferably in the treatment room. Some medication, such as eye drops, should be refrigerated. It is not good practice to store such medication in a refrigerator in the kitchen, the treatment room should be equipped with a small fridge where medication can be stored.

Medication for external use such as lotions and creams should not be stored with medicines for internal use such as tablets and syrups. They are usually stored in a cupboard in the treatment room. The storage of controlled drugs is governed by the Misuse of Drugs (Safe Custody) Regulations 1973[2]. Controlled drugs must be stored in a specially purchased metal cupboard designed for their storage.

Administration of drugs

Homes should have written policies regarding the administration of drugs. Written policies safeguard individual patients and nurses and reduce the possibility of errors occurring. At one time most hospitals insisted that two nurses carried out drug rounds, one dispensing medication whilst the other checked it and administered it. It is now common practice in many hospitals for one nurse to administer medication. This increases the possibility of error and in a nursing home environment, where many individuals require help to take their medication, makes administration much slower. Nurses within homes should discuss and decide policy on medication administration; it will depend on the size of the home and the numbers of trained staff on duty at any one time. Some homes have policies which state that whenever possible medication should be administered by two trained nurses, but when staffing levels or workload make this impractical medication may be dispensed by one trained nurse.

Second level nurses and drug administration

UKCC guidance[3] states that second level nurses should not administer medication unless under the direction of a first level registered nurse. Second level nurses may dispense medication in certain circumstances, and they must have additional instruction relevant to the medications they are likely to dispense in their current work area. An assessment is carried out to ensure that their theoretical knowledge of medication and their competency are adequate.

Unacceptable practices

Nurses in many settings will encounter registered nurses who dispense medications into medicine pots and place the individual's name on the pot. Several individual's medications are dispensed at once and all are placed on a tray. The nurse then carries the tray around and gives out the medication. This practice is known as secondary dispensing and is in contravention of UKCC guidelines. It is extremely dangerous – the possibilities of medication error are enormous – and is totally unacceptable. Written drug policies for the home should make it absolutely clear that this is forbidden.

Nurses should not alter labels. Wrongly labelled medication should be returned to the pharmacy. Nurses should not transfer medication from one container to another.

Identifying patients

Patients admitted to hospitals are given wrist bands showing their name and hospital number. In nursing homes the emphasis is on providing nursing care in a homely domestic environment and the use of name bands for identification purposes is rare. Usually the residents are well known to staff working at the home but occasionally agency or bank staff who are unfamiliar with all the patients are called upon to give out medication. The use of a photograph fixed to the drug chart enables nurses to identify individuals without resorting to institutional devices such as name bands.

Drug charts

Nurses are required to keep a record of all medication given. Normally medication is written up on a drug chart. In many homes nurses transcribe on to the chart the prescription written on an FP10 prescription by the individual's GP, and the doctor signs this chart. It is possible to buy ready-printed medication charts but nurses can have their own charts printed especially for their home (or group of homes) for little more than the cost of buying pre-printed charts. Many pre-printed charts run for 90 day cycles without requiring re-writing. This discourages regular medication reviews by doctors. It is good practice to use charts which require re-writing every 28–30 days. A sample chart is shown in Fig. 4.1.

Medication charts should have space to record drugs not given, the reasons for their omission, time, and the signature of the nurse. They should also have a separate section for 'as required' prescriptions; this should have sufficient space for nurses to indicate the time of administration and, if appropriate, the dose given. The chart should also have a section for 'once only' medications such as vaccinations. The sample chart (Fig. 4.1) also has a space labelled pharmacy. This space is used by nurses to record the date a new bottle of medication is commenced and how many tablets were in the bottle when it was opened. This is explained in detail in the drug auditing section later in this chapter.

Recording medication

It is essential that nurses maintain records of medication given. Medicine charts and patient records should be maintained for eight years after patient discharge or death. Medications are prescribed on a regular or 'as required' basis. Nurses should never give medication with which they are unfamiliar; they should look up the drug in an up to date version of the British National Formulary (BNF) or another reference book. Retail pharmacists are usually happy to supply complementary copies of the most up to date versions of these books to nursing homes they supply with drugs.

The nurse has a duty to withhold prescribed medication if she feels it is unsafe or unwise to administer it. A nurse who encounters a higher than normal dose of medication, or a chart and bottle showing different

ALLERGIES

Name:

Age:

G.P.:

DATE & MONTH				

DRUG (Approved Name)

DOSE	ROUTE	START DATE	DURATION

SIGNATURE		CANCEL DATE	PHARM

ADDITIONAL INSTRUCTIONS

6
10
12
14
18
22
24

DRUG (Approved Name)

DOSE	ROUTE	START DATE	DURATION

SIGNATURE		CANCEL DATE	PHARM

ADDITIONAL INSTRUCTIONS

6
10
12
14
18
22
24

DRUG (Approved Name)

DOSE	ROUTE	START DATE	DURATION

SIGNATURE		CANCE	PHARM

ADDITIONAL INSTRUCTIONS

6
10
12
14
18
22
24

DRUG (Approved Name)

DOSE	ROUTE	START DATE	DURATION

SIGNATURE		CANCEL DATE	PHARM

ADDITIONAL INSTRUCTIONS

6
10
12
14
18
22
24

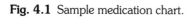

Fig. 4.1 Sample medication chart.

dosages, should withhold medication. The nurse who suspects that an individual is suffering an adverse drug reaction should withhold medication. In these circumstances the nurse should inform the patient's GP. She should record her reasons for withholding medication on the medication chart in the 'drugs not given section' and also in the nursing records. The nursing records should include details of any action she has taken such as returning medication to pharmacy or requesting that a doctor alter an incorrectly completed medication chart.

Controlled drugs

Controlled drugs should be recorded not only on the medication chart but also in the controlled drugs register. Controlled drugs registers can usually be purchased from the district pharmacist's office, which is usually based at the local hospital. A separate page is required for each medication. Two nurses should sign that they have checked and administered the prescribed medication. In small homes where only one registered nurse is on duty on a shift it is often possible for drug administration times of regular medications to coincide with handovers so that two nurses are available. If this is not possible, perhaps because medication is being given on an 'as required' basis, the registered nurse should ask a nursing auxiliary to check and sign that she has witnessed the registered nurse administering the medication to the patient. This is not a legal requirement but such practice protects both the patient and the nurse.

Drug audits

Nurses should audit medication every 28 to 30 days. The interval will depend on the prescription cycle in use by doctors who are providing medical care to older people within the home. In many homes one doctor cares for the majority of residents but in others there are a number of doctors. It is much easier if all doctors use the same prescription cycle and this can usually be arranged.

Auditing at first appears to involve a lot of hard work and the first reaction of some nurses is to think that it is creating work for work's sake. Auditing has two main functions; it enables nurses to monitor the usage of drugs and to ensure that they are being given correctly. It also ensures that each patient has sufficient drugs to carry them through a prescription cycle. This saves a lot of time and effort and with efficient auditing systems drugs do not run out, nurses do not have to constantly re-order drugs, and pharmacists do not have to keep rushing up and down to the home with prescription items. Auditing systems quickly repay the time and effort involved in setting them up.

When nurses have worked out the prescription cycle they will use they need to draw up a table of audit dates, medication order dates and delivery dates. The interval between the order date and delivery date should be discussed with the pharmacist. It is sensible to allow a week or ten days between order and delivery dates.

Pharmacists should be involved in drug audits whenever possible. In some circumstances the pharmacist cannot take part in every audit but should be involved in as many as possible. The pharmacist supplies a printed or typed list which gives details of each individual in the home and the name, dosage and frequency of each medication including details of 'as required' medication. The nurse and pharmacist check that the list and medication charts are identical and that there have been no recent changes which are not included on the pharmacist's list. Each regular medicine is counted and nurse and pharmacist ensure that there is sufficient medication until the next delivery date.

A note of the amount of medication required for the next prescription interval is put on the printout. This will usually be the same amount but it can vary. In some cases the amount of tablets prescribed has been reduced and a lesser amount can be ordered for the next prescription cycle. This eliminates waste. In other cases an individual has been admitted to hospital during a prescription cycle and so all medication prescribed has not been used and the hospital have usually provided a further two weeks' supply of medication on discharge. Medication prescribed on an 'as required' basis can either be counted or estimated depending on usage. This skill is rapidly acquired. Individuals admitted during a prescription cycle have their medication counted and sufficient is ordered to bring them in line with the prescription cycle.

Auditing enables pharmacist and nurse to compile a prescription list which is accurate and reflects the amount of medication required during the cycle. This is then entered on computer so that the pharmacist can keep accurate records of each individual's drug usage. A copy of the list, or the relevant sections relating to the individuals on a doctor's list, is sent to the doctor. The nurse and pharmacist retain a copy of the list, which can be posted, faxed or delivered to the home by the pharmacist. A copy of all prescriptions is then written into the drug ordering book by the nurse and checked by another nurse to ensure accuracy. The doctor(s) then issue individual prescriptions which are sent to the nursing home where they are checked for accuracy, stamped and collected by the pharmacist. This system has a number of checks which minimize the possibility of error.

The process of auditing sounds daunting and time consuming but once the system is in place the nurse and pharmacist can complete an audit on an average 39 bed nursing home in under two hours and it saves countless time over the prescribing period.

Avoiding auditing pitfalls

Changes of medication or dosage during a prescription cycle can cause problems with auditing. If a medication is prescribed during a prescription cycle, the amount of medication required to last until the next delivery date should be calculated. The doctor is then asked to prescribe this amount. The normal amount for the cycle is then ordered on the ordering date. When medication is increased the additional amount required until the next delivery cycle must be calculated and ordered. Short courses of medication such as antibiotics can be ordered as a complete course regardless of prescription cycle as they will not cause auditing problems. It is acceptable to order variable dose medications, such as warfarin or steroids, which are being reduced in amounts greater than the cycle, as the additional medication enables doctors to prescribe as clinically indicated without necessitating frequent calls to pharmacy. The drug audit will enable the nurse and pharmacist to check that the individual's stock levels of variable dose medication are sufficient.

Effective auditing is dependent on the nurse and pharmacist working together. It is essential that the nurse is able to rely on a cooperative professional pharmacist if the system is to function effectively.

Keeping records of medication entering the home

Details of all medication ordered and received should be kept in a bound book, giving details of the date of order, name of patient, drug, dosage and amount ordered. When medication is received this should be checked, either by the pharmacist and the nurse or two nurses, against the order; any discrepancies or shortfalls should be noted and both should sign. This book should contain details of any medication brought from hospital or home by individuals or supplied by doctors in an emergency situation. Failure to record all sources of medication will make auditing impossible.

Dealing with medication no longer required

Using a drug auditing system reduces excess stock within homes, but there are occasions when the nurse is left with medication which is no longer required. Discontinued medication should be returned to pharmacy. The medication of deceased patients should also be returned to pharmacy. It is recommended that nurses should remove medication for deceased patients from the medicine trolley, place it all in a container with a note stating the date of death, and lock this in a medicine cupboard. It should not be returned to pharmacy until seven days after the individual's death, in case the coroner should wish to have the medication examined. A record of all medication returned to pharmacy should be kept. This should be a bound book which should state the date, individual's name, name of medication, dose, amount returned and reason for returning to pharmacy. The nurse returning medication and the pharmacist receiving the medication should check these details together and should both sign the register of returned medications. There is no legal requirement to do this but it is good practice and ensures that every item of medication entering and leaving the home can be accounted for.

Medication review

All medications have adverse effects and for every benefit a drug offers there is also the risk of adverse reactions. These can have a profound effect on an older person's quality of life. It is policy on some elderly care units for doctors to discontinue all medication, monitor patient condition carefully and prescribe only when absolutely necessary. Some older adults, though, move through the health care system acquiring more medications as doctors treat them symptomatically. Older people are more likely to suffer from adverse reactions from medication because their renal and hepatic systems are less efficient and drugs remain in the system for longer. Nurses can encourage doctors to review medications regularly to ensure that older people are not prescribed medications which they no longer require. Nursing practice can have an important influence on the type of medication prescribed and the amount used.

Hypnotics

The use of hypnotics is widespread in nursing homes and research indicates that 33% to 45% of patients regularly receive night sedation[4, 5]. Hypnotics decrease the level of awareness and increase the risk of nocturia. Reduced ability to metabolize drugs rapidly can prolong drug half lives and the older person may be less alert during the day increasing the risk of incontinence[6]. Reduced levels of alertness can reduce mobility and muscle strength and can reduce diet and fluid intake, causing the older person to become weaker. These changes increase the risks of developing infection and pressure sores.

Nurses can encourage doctors to prescribe hypnotics on an 'as required' basis and can use nursing measures to enable older people to sleep well. In some units older people are assisted to bed by staff at around 7 PM. This discourages evening visits from friends and family. The need for sleep diminishes with age and it is quite normal for an older person to only require six or seven hours sleep. An older person who is asleep by 7 PM can be wide awake at 1 AM and nursing staff can report that insomnia is a problem and hypnotics can be prescribed. The real problem of course is nursing practice! Nurses can help ensure that older people sleep well without resorting to hypnotics.

Having realistic expectations about how much sleep an adult requires is the first step. Encouraging friends and relatives to visit even for a few minutes can help an older person go to bed happy and relaxed and more likely to have a good night's sleep. Encouraging older people to stay up later, perhaps watching a video, playing cards or reading a book will ensure that they go to bed when ready to sleep and not simply out of boredom. Bedrooms should be warm and comfortable. Offering hot milky drinks and ensuring night staff make minimal noise when moving around the home all help older people to sleep. Nurses who use their skills to help ensure older people are given a comfortable environment will find that they can virtually eliminate the use of hypnotics within the nursing home.

Diuretics

Nursing home patients are often prescribed diuretics; in one study 48% were on diuretic therapy[5], often for swollen ankles. Diuretic therapy can lead to urgency, frequency and urinary incontinence[7]. Urinary incontinence can be greatly reduced in nursing home patients if nursing staff treat postural oedema by encouraging exercise wherever possible, elevation of legs and the use of support stockings and tights. Diuretic therapy can, because of the fear of incontinence, cause elderly people to become less mobile and loss of mobility increases the risk of falls, leads to a reduction in muscle strength and increases the risk of the individual developing infection. The inappropriate use of diuretics can cause older people to become caught on a downward spiral of depression and loss of physical strength. Nursing intervention can successfully reduce or eliminate oedema and enable the use of diuretics to be greatly reduced.

Psychotropic drugs

Large numbers of nursing home patients (35–45%) are prescribed psychotropic drugs[8]. These reduce the level of alertness and individuals prescribed psychotropic drugs are at great risk of falling. Diet and fluid intake can be reduced due to drowsiness. Reduced alertness can also lead to incontinence. Nurses should encourage doctors to prescribe psychotropic drugs on an 'as required' basis and give them only as a last resort. The nurse can help older people who are unhappy and depressed by promoting an atmosphere within the home which enables people to maximize on their remaining abilities rather than focusing on disabilities; more information is given in Chapter 12. The nurse can help an older person more by listening and spending time discovering what is bothering the individual, rather than dispensing psychiatric drugs. Good nursing practice can significantly reduce the use of psychotropic medication within the nursing home.

Muscle relaxants

Muscle relaxants such as dantrolene and baclofen are frequently pre-scribed to treat spasticity following strokes. They frequently relax the urethral sphincter and lead to urinary incontinence. Exercise and passive movements can often effectively treat spasticity without adverse effects on continence. Relatives and friends can work with nursing staff to encourage these exercises and movements.

Anti-hypertensives

Anti-hypertensives can affect continence. They can lead to postural hypotension which can lead to falls, and these and the fear of falling can lead to loss of mobility and incontinence. Hypertension may be improved by gentle weight loss. Individuals prescribed hypotensives should have their blood pressure monitored regularly.

Summary

Older people are more likely to be prescribed a number of drugs than younger people and are at greater risk of suffering from adverse reac-tions to them than younger people. GPs are busy and do not always have time to review the need for medications. Nurses can influence the amount of drugs used within a nursing home and by working in part-nership with the older people and by using their nursing skills, they can ensure that older people are not prescribed medication unnecessarily.

Dealing with drug errors

Any nurse who makes or discovers a drug error has a duty to report that error. When a manager is informed that an error has occurred the individual's doctor should be informed immediately. The home should have a written policy which outlines action to be taken in such cir-cumstances. It is important for the manager to discover the reasons the error occurred and wherever possible to change practice to avoid such errors occurring in the future. The UKCC has expressed concern that nurses who have made mistakes under pressure of work and have reported such errors are subject to disciplinary action[9].

The use of disciplinary action in such circumstances may discourage nurses from reporting drug errors. It is important that the home's policy is just and fair and that the manager carefully considers the circumstances, and advises, counsels, identifies training needs and changes practice within the home if necessary. Disciplinary action will not rectify problems associated with busy periods of the day when nursing staff feel pressurized to complete the medication round as quickly as possible, but rearranging work patterns will help avoid future errors.

Conclusion

The nurse should be aware of the effects of medication and should inform the patient's doctor if an individual is suffering from side effects from medication. She can remind doctors to review medication regularly and can advise on its effectiveness. The use of a drug audit enables the nurse to check all medication which is brought to the home and detect errors in administration. Written policies on drug ordering, administration, disposal and the procedure to be followed if an error occurs protect patient and nurse.

Useful addresses and telephone numbers

Retail pharmacist   *District pharmacist*

References

(1) *Professional Conduct – Occasional Report on Standards of Nursing in Nursing Homes* (1994) UKCC, London.
(2) *Misuse of Drugs (Safe Custody) Regulations.* (1973) HMSO, London.
(3) *UKCC Standards for the Administration of Medicine.* (1992) UKCC, London.
(4) Hatton, P. (1990) Primum non nocere – an analysis of drugs prescribed to elderly patients in private nursing homes registered with Harrogate Health Authority. *Care of the Elderly*, April, **2**, (4) 166–8.
(5) Primrose W.R., Cappell, A.E., Simpson, G.E. *et al.* (1986) Prescribing patterns in registered nursing homes and long stay wards. *Age & Ageing*, 16, 25–8.
(6) Brocklehurst, J.C. (1984) Drug effects in urinary incontinence. In *Urology in the Elderly.* (ed. J.C. Brocklehurst), Churchill Livingstone, London.
(7) Kirkulata, G.H. (1981) Urinary incontinence secondary to drugs. *Urology*, 18, 618–19.
(8) Humphries, H.I. & Kassab, J.Y. (1986) An investigation into private sector nursing and residential homes for the elderly in North Wales. *Journal of Royal College of General Practitioners*, 36, 500–3.
(9) *UKCC Standards for the Administration of Medicine* (1992) paragraphs 41–43. UKCC, London.

Chapter 5
Infection Control

Introduction

The risks of acquiring an infection in hospital have been recognized for many years. Hospitals employ infection control nurses and have set up policies and procedures to reduce these risks and protect patients. Hospitals have policies which give guidance on procedures such as handwashing, dealing with infected and foul linen, and disposal of incontinence pads, soiled dressings and sharps. Nurses working in nursing homes may find that such policies do not exist in their work place. There is thought to be little need for infection control measures because nursing homes are not hospitals and there is little risk of infection in nursing homes. Such thoughts are understandable because little has been written about infection control in nursing homes and few homes have a full set of policies to prevent infection. Registration officers seldom enquire about infection control policies and infection rates within nursing homes are not monitored.

Infection risks in nursing homes

Older people are at risk of acquiring infection, and if they do it can lead to a decline in health, hospital admission and in some cases death[1]. The immune system becomes less effective in most adults as they age, so older adults are more at risk of acquiring infections than younger people[2]. Many older people living in nursing homes are extremely prone to infection, and research has identified a number of factors which increase the risk. Many older people living in nursing homes have conditions which predispose them to infection, and they are mal-nourished and so more likely to acquire infection. Providing a balanced diet and correcting malnutrition eliminates this risk[2]. Further information on nutrition is given in Chapter 10.

Individuals who suffer from urinary incontinence are likely to be referred for nursing home care[3], and these people are at risk of developing urinary tract infections[4]. Restoring continence using continence promotion strategies will eliminate this risk. Further information on continence promotion is given in Chapter 4.

Many older people are admitted to nursing homes with indwelling urinary catheters; older people who have urinary catheters normally develop urinary tract infections within seven days of catheterization. It is almost impossible to clear these infections whilst the catheter remains *in situ*[5] and catheterized individuals are at risk of ascending urinary tract infection[6]. In some cases it is possible to remove catheters and use continence promotion policies to restore continence, but in other cases catheterization is indicated. The use of long term catheters should be kept to a minimum to reduce infection risks. Older people who have long term catheters *in situ* can benefit from drinking two glasses of cranberry juice each day. Cranberry juice reduces infection by preventing bacteria from adhering to the mucosa in the urinary tract[7].

Older people who have just come out of hospital are at risk of developing an infection. Most older people are admitted to nursing homes from hospital, and those who have had operations recently are particularly at risk of developing infections; usually the more major the operation the greater the risk of infection. Nurses should observe such individuals for signs of infection. Individuals who share rooms are more at risk of acquiring infection than those nursed in single rooms.

How to assess risks

It is clear that some individuals are at great risk of developing an infection. Infection can be life threatening, and older people who do recover from infection often fail to make a full recovery and their quality of life is affected. Nurses have a legal duty under the Health & Safety at Work Act 1975[8] and a professional duty under the United Kingdom Central Council (UKCC) code of professional conduct to 'safeguard the interests and well-being of patients and clients'.

Assessment enables a nurse to discover which patients are at risk and to adopt a problem solving approach, preventing infection and minimizing risk. Risk assessment sounds like hard work – more paperwork and even less time to spend with patients. But it can be carried out quickly using a simple assessment form which has been designed specially for nursing home patients (Fig. 5.1). A few minutes spent assessing risk and planning care will prevent many patients from suffering infections that were preventable and will save nursing time. Prevention really is better than cure and nurses who assess risk and take action to reduce risks are able to control their workload and rarely find themselves having to react to a crisis.

Introducing policies and practices to reduce risks

All staff employed in nursing homes have an important role to play in preventing infection. Bacteria thrive in dirty and dusty conditions and high standards of cleanliness prevent infection. Domestic staff are important members of the team and the nurses should ensure that they are valued and feel that their role is appreciated. Staff who feel that their work is important and valued are motivated and their work is of a higher standard than the work of those who feel they are 'just the cleaner'.

Disposal of waste

Safe disposal of waste plays an important part in preventing infection. It is easier to ensure that waste is disposed of properly if written policies exist which inform staff how to dispose of waste. Nurses have a duty to ensure correct disposal of waste under the Environmental Protection Act 1990. Different types of waste should be stored in colour coded bags and dealt with in different ways.

Domestic waste

Domestic waste can be stored in black plastic bags. These are normally emptied into domestic dustbins in smaller homes, and in larger homes into large bins designed for commercial waste, such as Paladin bins which are normally supplied by the local council. Domestic waste is normally collected by the local council and arrangements can be made to have waste collected weekly or daily on weekdays. Nursing homes are classified as businesses and the council charges a fee for each bin emptied. Many homes have large amounts of waste and having it collected can be expensive. Some homes purchase compacters which compact waste and reduce the number of collections required.

Glass, broken crockery and aerosols

Glass, broken crockery and aerosols should be stored in a cardboard box and placed in a separate bin (usually a domestic dustbin) which has 'Glass' painted on it.

Clinical waste

Clinical waste should be collected and stored in yellow plastic bags. Clinical waste includes incontinence pads, and many homes have large amounts. Clinical waste is not collected with domestic waste, but in a separate vehicle. Many councils run a clinical waste collection service and arrange to have the waste collected once or twice a week, with a nominal charge of 50p or £1 per sack. Many nursing homes have great problems in storing volumes of clinical waste, and council clinical waste services were often designed as a service for local doctors' and dentists'

Infection risk assessment. The higher the sore the greater the risk of the patient developing an infection.

		Scores				
		0	1	2	3	4
Age:		☐	☐			
74 to 84	= 1					
85+	= 2					
Nutritional status:		☐	☐	☐	☐	
Normal	= 0					
Obese	= 1					
Thin	= 2					
Emaciated	= 3					
		☐	☐	☐		
Feeds self	= 0					
Poor appetite	= 1					
Dependent on nursing staff	= 2					
Continence status:		☐	☐	☐	☐	☐
Continent	= 0					
Urinary incontinence	= 1					
Urinary sheath	= 2					
Urinary catheter	= 3					
Faecally incontinent	= 4					
Skin integrity:		☐	☐	☐	☐	☐
Intact skin	= 0					
Skin ulcer (dependent on size/depth)	= 1 to 4					
Pressure sore (dependent on size/depth)	= 1 to 4					
Hospital admission/ treatment:		☐	☐	☐	☐	☐
Hospital admission within last 28 days	= 1					
Minor surgery (e.g. cataract)	= 2					
Major surgery (e.g. repair of fractured femur)	= 4					
Chemotherapy/ radiotherapy	= 4					
Medication:						
Steroid therapy	= 2			☐		
Antibiotic therapy	= 2			☐		
Sedatives	= 2			☐		

		Scores				
		0	1	2	3	4
Social factors:						
Sharing a room	= 1		☐			
Sharing with a catheterized patient	= 2			☐		
Sharing with a faecally incontinent patient	= 2			☐		
Sharing with a patient with skin lesion	= 2			☐		
Mobility:		☐	☐	☐	☐	☐
Mobile	= 0					
Mobile with help	= 1					
Wheelchair bound	= 2					
Immobile	= 3					
Bedfast	= 4					
Smoking:		☐		☐		
No	= 0					
Yes	= 2					
Total score	=					

Fig. 5.1 Infection control assessment form.

surgeries and were not designed to cope with the large volumes of incontinence pads which some homes can generate.

If local council services cannot cope, nurses can organize alternative means of disposal. Private companies offer special bins and clinical waste collection services, but these are expensive. The costs of collecting clinical waste from a typical 39 bed nursing home with an incontinence rate of 60% would be around £400 to £500 per month.

Pads can be incinerated but the Environment Protection Act 1990 specifies that the incinerator must reach extremely high temperatures and must satisfy stringent emission controls. The local council must also grant a licence before any incinerator can be used. Incinerators which meet such standards normally cost more than £10 000 and are beyond the means of most homes.

Pads can be broken up into a pulp in a macerator and pumped into the drains. A macerator offers a practical solution for many homes and the cost, usually £1000 to £1500, is quickly recovered. Homes must have a licence from the waste treatment and sewage department of the local water authority, which allows them to discharge macerator waste into the local sewage system. This licence normally costs a nominal amount, around £15 to £20, and is renewed annually. Soiled dressings, latex gloves, colostomy bags and disposable items such as catheters and catheter bags cannot be disposed of in macerators. Macerator blades get fouled up on such items.

The use of a macerator significantly reduces the amount of clinical waste, and council services or private contractors can be used to dispose of any remaining clinical waste. This is normally reduced to one or two bags per week. This clinical waste should be stored in yellow bags in dirty areas such as sluices. It should *never* be stored in clinical areas, patient areas or clean areas.

Sharps

Sharps such as lancets, syringes, needles, stitch cutters and any other item likely to pierce the skin cannot be placed in a yellow bag. They should be stored in a sharps bin, which should be placed in treatment rooms. In some cases a sharps bin can be stored in an individual's room. If a diabetic individual is receiving regular insulin injections and blood glucose monitoring, the risk of needlestick injuries can, in some cases, be reduced by placing a sharps box in the room. Nurses will have to balance this against the risk of the individual or other patients injuring themselves by investigating the sharps box.

It is possible to contract with private companies who will supply sharps bins and replace them at monthly, bi-monthly or quarterly intervals. This service normally costs between £30 and £60 per year depending on frequency. All companies supply spares so that bins do not become overfull, and they will change bins on request.

Dealing with linen

Many homes have their own laundries and employ staff to launder bedding, towels and patients' clothing. It is important to set out clear, written policies for storage of and cleaning linen.

All used linen should be stored in either clear plastic bags or white bags which are used specially for laundry. Soiled linen should be placed in red bags. It is possible to buy special bags with an alginate strip. These bags are placed in washing machines on a special sluice cycle, the alginate strip dissolves on contact with water, and the bag opens. The sluice cycle removes soiling and at the end of the cycle the alginate bag is disposed of and the linen is washed in the machine. The use of alginate bags ensures that soiled linen is handled only once and this reduces the risk of infection. Staff handling soiled linen should wear an apron and gloves. Hands should be washed after the gloves and apron have been removed.

Items such as table cloths should be washed separately from bed linen or clothing. Ensuring that the home is kept clean, that waste is disposed of appropriately and that linen is stored appropriately and laundered correctly ensures that environmental hazards are reduced and basic safeguards are in place. Nurses can then go on to introduce specific measures to reduce infection within nursing homes.

Universal precautions

The single most important action staff can do to prevent infection is to wash their hands before and after attending to each patient. Bacteria are normally transferred from patient to patient on the unwashed hands of care givers[9]. The importance of handwashing and its role in preventing cross infection cannot be overemphasized.

Homes should provide facilities to ensure correct handwashing techniques. Handwashing facilities should be provided in treatment rooms, sluices, toilets, bathrooms and other areas. Wash-basins should have taps which can be operated using wrists or elbows. Disposable paper towels should be used to dry hands. A foot operated bin should be provided for disposal of used towels. Liquid soap in wall mounted dispensers should be used; perfumed soaps and soaps containing lanolin should be avoided as these can cause allergies and dermatitis in some individuals.

When staff should wash their hands

- at the beginning of each shift
- before serving meals
- before giving out medications
- after handling laundry and making beds
- before physical contact with a patient
- after physical contact with a patient
- after removing aprons and gloves
- before, during, and after performing aseptic techniques
- at the end of each shift.

A laminated card detailing universal precautions is available free to members of the Royal College of Nursing. Their address is 20 Cavendish Square, London W1M 0AB.

Establishing protocols for suspected infection

Research from nursing homes in North America demonstrates that older people living in nursing homes are at risk of becoming infected with organisms which are resistant to many antibiotics normally prescribed. Doctors caring for older people living in nursing homes tend to prescribe antibiotics without sending specimens for culture and sensitivity tests[10]. While this practice might be appropriate for adults living in the community it is bad practice in nursing homes.

In many cases older people thought to be suffering from an infection are prescribed antibiotics by doctors who fail to carry out physical examinations. One research study checked if infection was present when doctors had prescribed antibiotics and if organisms cultured were sensitive to the antibiotic prescribed. This study revealed that only just over half of the antibiotics prescribed were indicated and appropriate[11]. Older people in nursing homes run the risk of being prescribed antibiotics unnecessarily and can suffer from unpleasant side effects. Other older people suffering from infections which can be life threatening[1] are treated with antibiotics which will not improve their condition.

Nurses can work with doctors to establish protocols which reduce the risk of older people receiving inappropriate or unnecessary antibiotics.

A protocol on wound infection should include information about wound healing and the action of dressings and the fact that when using some dressings such as hydrocolloids odour is not necessarily indicative of infection. Nurses and doctors can agree a procedure which nurses can follow if a wound infection is suspected. This will normally include checking an individual's temperature, pulse, respirations and blood pressure and sending a wound swab for culture and sensitivity. Doctors are informed of the nurse's action and may wish to commence treatment with antibiotics without awaiting the results of the wound swab if they feel such action is clinically indicated. In most cases doctors will await the result of the wound swab and prescribe antibiotics if these are indicated.

A protocol on suspected chest infection would follow a similar format and sputum specimens would be sent for culture and sensitivity testing whenever possible. A protocol on suspected urinary tract infection would include sending a urine specimen.

Establishing written protocols to deal with cases of suspected infection can reduce antibiotic usage dramatically within nursing homes and can improve the quality of care[12].

Monitoring infections

Keeping records of the number of infections within the home, the individuals affected, the site of the infection, the investigations undertaken, treatment and outcome is important. These records enable nurses to detect infections and to take appropriate nursing action to prevent cross infection. Infection control records can be completed quickly using a simple form. An example is shown in Fig. 5.2.

Date, Name and Number	Site of infection and type of infection (i.e. wound/urine)	Clinical symptoms (i.e. pyrexial, etc.)	Investigations carried out by nursing staff (i.e. blood pressure, temperature)	Type of swab or specimen sent and date (i.e. wound and sputum)	Swab results and treatment recommended by doctor	Review of treatment and date

Fig. 5.2 Infection control monitoring form.

Preventing cross infection is always important but extra vigilance is required when individuals are harbouring multi-resistant bacteria such as methicillin resistant staphylococcus aureus.

Methicillin resistant staphylococcus aureus

Introduction

Methicillin resistant staphylococcus aureus (MRSA) has caused outbreaks of infection in UK hospitals since the 1980s. There is evidence to suggest that the prevalence of MRSA has been increasing in southern England since 1986[13]. Older adults resident in nursing homes are at risk of contracting MRSA infection. Nursing home staff fear that if they accept new residents with MRSA they will be placing their existing residents at risk[14]. Many nursing homes will not admit MRSA positive individuals. Some nursing home proprietors have been informed by their insurers that if they knowingly admit an individual with MRSA they risk having their insurance cover voided. Some social services departments have informed nurses that they will refuse to place any patients in homes where there is a known case of MRSA. Nurses in homes have no firm guidance about the risks MRSA poses in nursing homes or their role in preventing the spread of MRSA whilst enabling the older adults colonized or infected with MRSA to lead normal lives.

Epidemiology – what is MRSA?

Methicillin resistant staphylococcus aureus (MRSA) is a methicillin resistant strain of staphylococcus aureus, which is a common bacterium. Staphylococcus aureus are nonspore-forming gram positive cocci which appear as golden tinged clusters when seen under a microscope[15]. Resistant strains of staphylococcus aureus developed shortly after the introduction of antibiotics in 1941[16]. This is illustrated in Table 5.1[17].

Table 5.1 Development of resistant strains of staphylococcus aureus.

Date antibiotic introduced	Resistance identified
Penicillin 1941	1940s
Streptomycin 1944	mid 1940s
Tetracycline 1948	1950s
Erythromycin 1952	1950s
Methicillin 1959	late 1960s
Gentamycin 1964	mid 1970s

There are many strains of staphylococcus aureus but they can be considered as four main groups (Table 5.2).

Table 5.2 Four main groups of strains of staphylococcus aureus.

(1) Penicillin sensitive strains.
(2) Penicillin resistant; sensitive to methicillin and cephalosporins.
(3) 'Borderline' resistant strains sensitive to methicillin.
(4) MRSA resistant to methicillin and cephalosporins. Most strains of MRSA are also resistant to erythromycin, clindamycin, tetracycline and aminoglycocides[18, 19].

Transmission of MRSA

MRSA is rarely spread by airborne transmission[20]. There is little evidence to suggest that nasal carriers of MRSA transmit disease[20], but despite this there have been attempts to eradicate MRSA in nasal carriers. Attempts to eradicate MRSA in colonized individuals have been found to be not only unnecessary and ineffective but also potentially hazardous because MRSA strains isolated after attempted eradication had acquired resistance to even more antibiotics[21]. MRSA is normally spread from patient to patient on the hands of nursing and medical staff[22]. The length of time it remains on the hands varies from minutes to hours[23, 24]. MRSA can be removed by washing hands thoroughly with soap and water[25].

Colonization or infection?

Many individuals are colonized with staphylococcus aureus. Research indicates that 40% of adults demonstrate nasal carriage of methicillin sensitive staphylococcus aureus[18]. Many individuals are colonized with staphylococcus aureus but have no evidence of disease. Nursing home residents, in common with the general population, are colonized with a number of bacteria including staphylococcus aureus[19]. It is important that the nurse ascertains if an individual is colonized or infected with MRSA (Table 5.3) as this will affect the infection control measures required.

Who is at risk of contracting MRSA infection?

MRSA is not a danger for healthy individuals. Staff caring for patients are not at risk and they will not carry the infection home and put their families at risk. Visitors, including pregnant women, babies and young children, are not at risk. In nursing homes only patients who have

Table 5.3 Presence of MRSA.

Infection	Colonization
Bacteria present	Bacteria present
Pyrexia	Apyrexial
Signs of infection e.g. wound infection, chest infection, urinary tract infection	No signs of infection
Appears unwell	Appears well

urethral or suprapubic catheters, nasogastric or gastrostomy tubes, tracheostomy, leg ulcers, pressure sores or are extremely frail, are at risk[26].

Preventing the spread of MRSA in nursing homes

The number of individuals with MRSA in UK nursing homes is unknown. It has been suggested that many suffer from undetected MRSA infection and that their re-admission to hospitals perpetuates a cycle of infection[27]. North American research indicates high levels of MRSA in nursing homes and the spread of MRSA within these homes is attributed to inadequate knowledge of infection control strategies, and poor nursing practice[28]. The introduction of an infection control programme will enable nursing staff to determine which bacteria are causing infection within their nursing home and to use appropriate strategies to prevent cross infection[29].

Preventing the spread of infection

The most important aspect of preventing the spread of MRSA is handwashing. Each time a member of the nursing staff attends to a patient they should wash their hands with soap and water and dry them with a paper towel. Some practitioners advocate the use of chlorhexidine hand disinfectant followed by the use of a chlorhexidine alcohol hand rub, but further research is required into the necessity and cost effectiveness of this policy[30]. The routine use of hand disinfections and alcohol rubs can cause hands to become very dry and cracked, which makes them at risk of becoming infected with MRSA; so such strategies may well lead to further outbreaks of MRSA.

Some practitioners recommend the use of latex gloves when touching colonized or infected patients. This practice could upset and alarm older adults. The use of latex gloves is not a substitute for handwashing. Gloves can give nurses a false sense of security and they may omit handwashing. Further research is required into the costs of latex gloves, their effectiveness and how using them at all times when touching MRSA infected or colonized individuals affects the patient's sense of well being. Latex gloves should be used when handling body secretions from individuals who are MRSA infected. Cuts or areas of broken skin on a nurse's hands should be covered with an occlusive waterproof dressing.

Caring for MRSA infected wounds

Wounds infected with MRSA should be covered with an occlusive waterproof dressing which effectively contains exudate. A strict aseptic technique should be used. The nurse should wear latex gloves and a disposable plastic apron which should be discarded after the dressing is completed. Ideally the nurse dressing this wound should not dress other patients' wounds. If this is not possible the MRSA infected wound should be dressed after all other dressings have been completed.

Can MRSA infected individuals share a room?

It is preferable to nurse MRSA infected individuals in single rooms. Many nursing homes have shared rooms and individuals may be sharing with a spouse or someone who has become a friend. It is possible to nurse MRSA infected individuals in shared rooms provided they meet the criteria in the next paragraph and strict infection control procedures are adhered to – this is shown in Table 5.4. One study found that there was a greater incidence of MRSA spread from individuals in single rooms than in shared rooms. The study, however, gives no details of infection control procedures within the nursing homes concerned[14].

The MRSA infected or colonized patient should be alert, able and willing to assist nursing staff in preventing MRSA spread, and should not

Table 5.4 Criteria for containment of MRSA.

MRSA in wound	An occlusive dressing effectively contains exudate
MRSA in sputum	The patient uses tissue or sputum pot to contain sputum
MRSA in urine	The patient is continent and uses toilet The patient has a catheter which is patent and there is no spillage of urine
MRSA in faeces	The patient is continent of faeces The patient has a stoma and stoma appliances effectively contain faeces without leakage

share a room with any individual who has a skin lesion, an indwelling catheter, nasogastric or gastrostomy tube or a tracheostomy, or is very frail, as such individuals are at risk of contracting MRSA infection[26, 28].

MRSA infected individuals who fulfil the criteria for room sharing can lead an unrestricted life both inside and outside the nursing home. They can take part in normal social activities and join others for meals in the dining room; there is no need to use disposable crockery or cutlery. They can go out to the shops or to visit their family. If nursing staff experience difficulty in containing infected sputum, wound exudate, urine or faeces they should contact the local infection control nurse for further advice.

Clothing and bedding

The infected individual's clothing and bedding should be treated as infected. Nursing staff should wear disposable plastic aprons and wash their hands thoroughly after handling clothing and bedding. Many homes now use water soluble bags for infected or soiled linen and clothing, which is washed separately.

Communication

An individual who is MRSA positive should have this recorded on their care plan. Infection control measures, actions, intentions and evaluation of care should be recorded.

If a visit to a hospital, perhaps for an outpatient's appointment, is planned, hospital staff should be notified of the individual's MRSA status prior to the appointment. Ambulance staff should also be notified. If the individual is attending the accident and emergency unit, staff should be informed of the MRSA status so that they can use appropriate infection control measures. Communication between hospital and nursing home is essential if the spread of MRSA is to be minimized. Hospital staff also have an important role to play in informing nursing home staff of a patient's MRSA status.

Conclusion

MRSA infected individuals may be safely cared for in nursing homes and can enjoy a good quality of life without compromising the safety of others if infection control measures and strategies for containment are applied. Nursing home staff should always enquire if individuals are colonized or infected with MRSA prior to arranging admission from hospital or community.

Further information and help

Infection control nurses are employed in community and hospital settings. Nurses working in nursing homes should enquire if there is a community based infection control nurse. If not, usually the hospital based infection control nurse will advise staff in nursing homes.

Nurses who wish to find out more about the role of infection control nurses can often arrange to spend a day with one locally. Some hospitals and colleges of nursing run study days on infection control and would welcome staff from nursing homes.

Useful addresses and telephone numbers

Infection control nurse

Microbiology Lab

References

(1) Irvine, P., Van Burren, N. *et al.* (1984) Causes of hospitalisation of nursing home residents: the role of infection. *Journal of the American Geriatric Society*, 32, 103–7.
(2) Chandra, R. (1989) Nutritional regulation of immunity and the risk of infection in old age. *Immunology*, 67, 141–7.
(3) Ouslander, J., Kane, R. *et al.* (1982) Urinary incontinence in elderly nursing home patients. *Journal of American Medical Association*, **248** (10) 1194–8.
(4) Brocklehurst, J., Dillane, J. *et al.* (1986) The prevelance and symptamology of urinary infection in an aged population. *Gerontologia Clinica*, 10, 242–53.
(5) Clifford, C. (1982) Urinary tract infection: a brief selective overview. *International Journal of Nursing Studies*, 19, 213–22.
(6) Platt, R., Polk, B. *et al.* (1983) Reduction of mortality associated with noscominal urinary tract infection. *New England Journal of Medicine*, 307, 637–42.

(7) Nazarko, L. (1995) Cranberry juice and prevention of urinary tract infections. *Nursing Standard*, in press.

(8) Health & Safety at Work Act (1975). HMSO, London.

(9) Cookson, B., Peters, B., Webster, M., Phillips, I., Rahman, M. & Noble, W. (1989) Staff carriage of epidemic methicillin resistant staphlococcus aureus. *Journal Clinical Microbiology*, 27, 1471–6.

(10) Zimmer, J., Bentley, D. *et al.* (1986) Systemic antibiotic use in nursing homes a quality assessment. *Journal American Geriatric Society*, 34, 703–10.

(11) Katz, P., Thomas, R. *et al.* (1990) Antibiotic use in nursing home patients, physician practice patterns. *Archives of Internal Medicine*, 150, 1465–8.

(12) Nazarko, L. (1994) Preventing infection in nursing homes. *Elderly Care*, **6** (4) 14–16.

(13) MacIntosh, C.A., Marples, R.R. & Kerr, G.E. (1991) Surveillance of MRSA in England & Wales 1986–90. *Journal Hospital Infection*, 18, 279–92.

(14) Beedle, D. (1993) Beating the bug. *Nursing Times, Journal of Infection Control Nursing* (supplement), **89** (45) 2–6.

(15) Morita, M. (1993) Methicillin resistant staphyloccus aureus, past, present and future. *Nursing Clinics of North America*, **28** (3) 625–37.

(16) Nue, H.C. (1992) The crisis in antibiotic resistance. *Science*, 257, 1064–73.

(17) Shanson, D.C. (1992) Antibiotic resistance in staphyloccus aureus. In *Methicillin Resistant Staphlococcus Aureus Clinical Management and Laboratory Standards* (ed. M.T. Cafferty). Marcel Dekker, New York.

(18) Waldvogel, F.A. (1990) Staphylococcus aureus. In *Principles and Practices of Infectious Diseases* (eds R.J. Douglas Jnr & J.E. Bennett). Churchill-Livingstone, Edinburgh.

(19) Boyce, J.M. (1991) Patterns and prevelance of methicillin resistant staphylococcus aureus. *Infection Control and Hospital Epidemiology*, **12** (2) 79–82.

(20) Boyce, J.M. (1992) Methicillin resistant staphyloccus aureus – detection, epidemiology and control measures. *Infection Control and Hospital Epidemiology*, 13, 725–37.

(21) Hsu, C.C.S. (1991) Serial survey of methicillin resistant staphyloccus aureus nasal carriage among residents in a nursing home. *Infection Control and Hospital Epidemiology*, **12** (7) 416–21.

(22) Thompson, R.L., Carbezudo, I. & Wenzel, R.P. (1982) Epidemiology of noscominal infections caused by methicillin resistant staphylococcus aureus. *Annals Internal Medicine*, 97, 309–17.

(23) Cookson, B., Peters, B., Webster, M. Phillips, I., Rahman, M. & Noble, W. (1989) Staff carriage of epidemic methicillin resistant staphylococcus aureus. *Journal Clinical Microbiology*, 27, 1471–6.

(24) Peacock, J.E. (jnr) Marsik, F.J. & Wenzel, R.P. (1980) Methicillin resistant staphyloccus aureus: introduction and spread within a hospital. *Annals Internal Medicine*, 93, 526–32.

(25) Crossley, K., Landesman, B. Zaske, D. (1979) An outbreak of infections caused by strains of staphyloccus aureus resistant to methicillin and aminoglcosides. *Journal Infectious Diseases*, 139, 280–7.

(26) O'Toole, R.D., Drew, W.I., Dahgren, B.J. & Beaty, H.N. (1970) An outbreak of methicillin resistant staphyloccus aureus infection: observations in hospital and nursing home. *Journal American Medical Association*, 213, 257–62.

(27) Goodall, B. & Tompkins, D.S. (1994) Nursing homes act as a reservoir. *British Medical Journal*, 308–58.

(28) Hsu, C.C.S., Malculuso, C.P., Special, L. & Hubble, R.H. (1988) High rate of methicillin resistant staphlococcus aureus isolates from hospitalised nursing home patients. *Archives of Internal Medicine*, 148, 569–70.

(29) Nazarko, L. (1994) Preventing infection in nursing homes. *Elderly Care*, **6** (4) 14–16.

(30) Tuffnell, D.J., Croton, R.S., Hemingway, D.M., Hartley, M.N., Wake, P.N. & Garvey, R.J.P. (1978) Methicillin resistant staphyloccus aueus; the role of antisepsis in the control of an outbreak. *Journal Hospital Infection*, 10, 255–9.

Chapter 6
Wound Care

Introduction

The commonest types of wounds cared for by nurses within nursing homes are leg ulcers and pressure sores (decubitus ulcers); fungating lesions and surgical wounds are less common. Wound care within nursing homes is generally the responsibility of the nurse. Leg ulcers in particular can be chronic and simply caring for the wound is not enough. Research indicates that individuals can suffer from recurrent leg ulcers over periods ranging from $10^{(1)}$ to 50 years[2]. Many nurses have seen leg ulcers heal only to see them break down again.

There has been a revolution in wound care in recent years and we now know more about the anatomy and physiology of wound healing than ever before. Research within nursing homes demonstrates that nurses use modern dressings such as hydrocolloids and alginates appropriately in the majority of cases and often go to considerable trouble to obtain dressings not currently available on FP10 prescription for individuals in nursing homes. Nurses report feeling isolated and find it difficult to obtain access to study days and courses dealing with wound care[3]. There are many articles in the nursing journals which provide guidance on choosing dressings but there are few which examine the underlying causes of leg ulcers and help nurses to treat the patient who has a leg ulcer, rather than simply the ulcer. This chapter aims to assist the nurse to provide holistic treatment for the individual with a chronic wound, and by correcting, wherever possible, factors which predispose to chronic wounds, to prevent tissue breakdown in the future.

The importance of assessment

Nurses have a duty under the UKCC code of conduct to ensure that their practice promotes and safeguards the wellbeing of patients. Nurses have a duty to remain professionally up to date and to work with patients to provide the best care possible. The nurse normally works out a plan of care, documents the nursing aims and intentions and after a period of time evaluates the effectiveness of the care she has given. Leg ulcers have various causes, and treatment which would be effective and promote healing with a leg ulcer of venous origin could prove disastrous when used on an ulcer of arterial or mixed venous and arterial origin. The nurse has a duty to discover the type of ulcer before she can begin treatment. Discovering the factors which contributed to the development of the ulcer and, wherever possible, eliminating them helps existing wounds to heal more rapidly and prevents their recurrence.

Many nurses recoil from the idea of yet more assessment and yet more paperwork. Real nurses want to spend time with their patient, not processing yet more paperwork. Assessment of an individual with a chronic wound is not a sterile exercise where the nurse retires to the office to tick boxes. Assessment can only be carried out by talking to and examining the patient, and gives the nurse a chance to really get to know the patient. By identifying the type of ulcer and the predisposing factors the nurse can work with the patient to solve the problems which caused the wound to become chronic. Assessment can save the nurse many unnecessary hours of dressing a wound that fails to heal because only the wound is being treated and not the person with the wound. A half hour spent assessing the person with a chronic wound can save the person weeks and months of suffering and the nurse countless hours of time. The time saved can be spent doing what all nurses wish to do – spending time with patients.

Aims of assessment

There are four aims of assessment.

(1) To find out what the patient feels the main problem is. This is the most important aspect of the assessment.

> Ethel Davis a 92 year old was admitted to a nursing home with gross oedema of the leg and a large heavily exuding leg ulcer. Ethel was extremely depressed and her appetite was poor. She explained to her assessing nurse that her greatest problem was that she could not wear her shoes because of the oedema. This prevented her walking a few steps from her daughter's car to a friend's house where she had played bridge weekly for over 40 years. The nurse organized a referral to the local orthotist who made special boots to accommodate the oedema. Ethel's depression resolved, her appetite improved and exercise combined with treatment to the ulcer resolved the oedema.

(2) The next aim of assessment is to discover what the patient hopes to achieve. What are the patient's aims?

> Victoria Bruce was suffering from a small arterial ulcer. It appeared almost insignificant when compared to the large

venous ulcers her assessing nurse had seen. This ulcer, however, was acutely painful and every night Mrs Bruce awoke in
excruciating pain which was only relieved when she dangled
her legs over the edge of the bed. Mrs Bruce had not had a
decent night's sleep in months. The assessing nurse was able to
ensure that Mrs Bruce received analgesia to relieve her pain
and ensured that this was given just before Mrs Bruce went to
sleep.

(3) The next aim of assessment is to identify the cause of the ulcer and
to discuss treatment with the patient. This is examined in detail later
in the chapter.
(4) The final aim of assessment is to identify the factors which have
contributed to the ulcer and to discuss and plan treatment with the
patient. This is also examined in detail later in the chapter.

Causes of leg ulcers

The incidence of leg ulcers rises with age. They occur in 3.6% of people
over the age of 65 and women over the age of 85 are ten times more
likely to develop them than men are. Leg ulcers on half of all individuals
have failed to heal within a year[4].

Venous ulcers

Venous ulcers are the most common type of leg ulcers (70% of the total)
and develop because valves in the deep and perforating veins become
incompetent. This leads to poor venous drainage from the legs and
chronic venous hypertension develops. Individuals with this hypertension normally have prominent varicose veins on their legs. They often
experience ankle swelling but rarely have marked oedema to the leg.
Infection should be suspected in individuals with marked oedema. The
individual may complain of itching over the veins.

Venous ulcers can be very large and are often oval in shape. They are
rarely painful unless there is marked oedema present or they are
infected. The individual with venous ulcers usually complains of aching
and a feeling of heaviness. This is relieved by elevating the feet. The skin
around the ulcer is often brown; this is known as staining and is caused
by leakage of blood into the capillaries just under the skin. Small dis-
tended veins can often be seen around the ankles.

Arterial ulcers

Arterial ulcers are less common than venous ulcers (10% of the total).
They are caused by arterial disease which can affect large or small
arterial vessels. Arterial disease affects blood supply to the leg. Indivi-

duals with arterial ulcers are more likely to be male. They may suffer from hypertension, diabetes or rheumatoid arthritis. The individual will have cold feet, the legs are usually hairless and the skin is pale and develops a shiny appearance. The feet are often a dusky pink. Pedal pulses are usually absent or very faint. Pedal pulses can be difficult to feel if oedema is present and it is best to confirm the absence of pedal pulses using a Doppler ultrasound. Ischaemic ulcers are normally very small and deep. They often have a punched out appearance and are irregular in shape. They can be extremely painful. The individual usually finds that the pain is relieved by dangling the legs over the edge of the bed. Elevating the leg causes it to become white, known as blanching, and causes pain.

Ulcers of mixed aetiolgy

Some individuals suffer from ulcers which have been caused by a mixture of arterial and venous disease.

Factors which influence wound healing

Wound healing is affected by factors which affect the wound and factors which affect the patient with the wound. An understanding of these factors is essential if nurses are to provide the optimum environment for wound healing to take place.

Ageing slows the rate of wound healing and the skin of older people is more prone to damage than that of younger people[5].

Drugs such as steroids and non steroidal anti-inflammatory drugs can impair healing by reducing the normal inflammatory response required in wound healing. The nurse should be aware of the possibility of tissue damage in such patients and should secure dressings with bandages or tubular bandages instead of tape wherever possible.

Long standing illness can affect the entire body and delay wound healing.

Diabetes can compromise circulation and hyperglycaemia can delay healing[6]. The presence of a wound, especially an infected wound, can lead to poor diabetic control and can further inhibit healing. Individuals suffering from diabetes who develop a leg ulcer require close monitoring of their blood glucose and may require additional medication to control diabetes because of the wound. It is essential to ensure that the diabetes is well controlled as high glucose levels will not only inhibit healing but also predispose to infection which will further destabilize diabetic control.

Iron deficiency and pernicious anaemia delay wound healing as haemoglobin is low. Low levels of haemoglobin reduce the body's ability to transport oxygen. Wounds require high levels of oxygen in order to heal; low levels of oxygen delay healing[7]. Iron deficiency anaemia is common in some older people who no longer have the energy or take the time and trouble to eat a balanced diet.

Many older people are prescribed either steroids or non steroidal anti-inflammatory drugs for arthritis. These drugs can cause gastric ulceration and gastric bleeding. This bleeding can be either acute or chronic, and chronic slow gastric bleeding can cause severe anaemia over a period of time. Pernicious anaemia is caused by a lack of an intrinsic factor and is treated with vitamin B12 injections. Treatment of anaemia will improve wound healing by increasing the amount of oxygen at the wound surface.

Cardiac disease impairs wound healing by reducing blood flow throughout the body. This reduces the oxygen and nutrients available to the wound. Treatment of cardiac disease often leads to more efficient cardiac output and this improves wound healing[5].

Hypertension leads to decreased blood flow to the wound and impairs healing. In obese individuals hypertension often resolves with weight loss. In some individuals medication is required. Treatment of hypertension improves wound healing

Thyroid disease The thyroid gland is responsible for controlling metabolic rate. An underactive thyroid gland (hypothyroidism) will slow down wound healing. Treatment with thyroxine will restore normal metabolic function and facilitate wound healing.

Nutrition and wound healing

Nutrition is one of the key factors in healing wounds. Healing is impaired in obese individuals because blood supply to adipose tissue is poor. This affects blood supply to the wound. Underweight individuals usually lack the protein reserves required to repair tissues. Both underweight and obese individuals normally have a poor diet and this affects the supply of nutrients available to the wound.

Individuals with wounds require a high calorie diet as healing increases the metabolic rate and additional calories are required to enable the body to repair damaged tissues. It is recommended that individuals with wounds have at least 2500 calories per day. The more extensive the wound the greater the individual's calorie requirement; in some cases as many as 5000 calories per day are required[5]. Individuals who do not consume sufficient calories initially utilize body fat stores and when these are exhausted begin to lose protein from muscle tissue. An adequate diet containing a mixture of carbohydrate, fat and protein is required if wounds are to heal. Carbohydrates provide energy for cell metabolism, fats are essential if cells are to regenerate and protein is required to enable a blood supply to be established to growing cells and to build collagen which is necessary for tissue repair.

Vitamins and trace elements

Vitamins and trace elements are required to enable wounds to heal. Vitamin A is required to repair tissues. Vitamin C is essential in wound repair and enables the body to fight infection. Vitamin B complex is required if cells are to reproduce. Vitamin K is required to enable blood clotting to take place and enable wounds to heal. Zinc deficiency delays wound healing[8]. It can be difficult to ensure that older adults consume a diet with sufficient calories and nutrients to enable optimal wound healing to take place. Many individuals with wounds will require dietary supplements to ensure an adequate diet. Many dietary supplements are available on prescription and contain a balance of fat, carbohydrate, protein and vitamins. A range of supplements are available, including ready-made puddings and drinks. Nurses who require advice on how to meet an individual's dietary requirements must ask the patient's doctor to make a referral to the local community or hospital based dietician. Nurses are unable to refer individuals direct to dieticians.

Importance of fluid intake

An adequate fluid intake of 1.5 to 2 litres per day is required in healthy adults. Individuals with heavily exuding wounds require higher than normal fluid intake. If fluid intake is not sufficiently high to compensate for exudate, the individual becomes dehydrated. Dehydration affects electrolyte balance and inhibits wound healing.

Mobility

Mobility plays an important part in wound healing. Individuals who are suffering from venous ulceration benefit from exercise which encourages venous drainage and reduces oedema. Individuals with ulcers of vascular origin benefit from gentle exercise which improves circulation. People who are immobile are more at risk of developing deep vein thrombosis and postural oedema than those who are mobile.

Factors which affect the wound

The aim of traditional wound care was to keep wounds clean, dry and free from bacteria. Wounds were cleaned daily with antiseptics and encouraged to dry out. Research has now proved that wounds heal best in a warm moist environment[9].

Cleaning wounds reduces their temperature below body temperature and this slows the rate of cellular repair[10]. Many cleansing agents have been proved to damage granulating wounds; these include Eusol[11], chlorhexidine, cetrimide[12] and providone iodine[13].

The use of gauze can damage healthy granulation tissue and impede healing[14].

It is apparent that nurses who are not aware of research findings on wound healing can impair the rate of wound healing by choosing the wrong dressing, cleaning wounds with disinfectants which will delay healing, or cleaning wounds unnecessarily and more frequently than required. Assessing the individual with a wound, taking a nursing history, and implementing and evaluating treatment will enable the nurse to provide modern research based care.

Nursing history and further investigations

The aim of the nursing history is to identify how the ulcer is affecting the individual's life and what the patient wishes to achieve. It is essential to identify the causes of the ulcer and the factors which contributed to the ulcer developing and are delaying healing.

The nurse should ask if the patient has ever had a fracture in the ulcerated leg. A history of previous fracture is common in individuals with venous ulceration. The nurse should enquire if there is any history of venous problems such as varicose veins, deep vein thrombosis or 'white leg of pregnancy' which is caused by venous occlusion. The nurse should record any previous treatment of venous problems such as injection or surgery. A history of cerebro-vascular accidents, transient ischaemic attacks, angina or mycardial infarction indicates arterial problems. Diabetes and rheumatoid arthritis also indicate possible arterial problems.

The history should include details of dietary and fluid intake. The individual's weight should be recorded, and they should be asked if there are any difficulties with walking.

The nurse should ask how long the wound has been present and how it has been treated. It may be necessary to obtain further information on previous wound care from community or hospital based nurses. Details of any wound investigations should be obtained. Urine should be checked for glucose.

The patient's doctor should be encouraged to order a full blood count if anaemia is suspected, thyroid function tests if hypothyroidism is suspected and serum albumen levels if gross oedema is present. If the wound is a chronic wound then patch testing for allergens may be indicated.

The use of Doppler ultrasound to record resting pressure index is valuable because pressures of more than 0.9 indicate venous disease and pressures of less than 0.9 indicate arterial disease. Doppler ultrasound readings can be carried out by doctors or nurses trained in this technique[15].

Assessing and measuring the wound

It is important to measure the wound as the nurse can then keep a record of healing. The usual method of measuring is to trace an outline of the wound on to a piece of plastic film with an indelible pen. The wound is measured at intervals and a record of progress can be kept.

Wounds are normally classified in five basic groups:

- necrotic – covered with a hard black necrotic area
- infected – red, inflamed, cellulitis present, odour
- yellow and sloughy – covered with soft yellow or white slough
- granulating – clean, pink/yellow
- epitheliasing – clean, pink/white, superficial

The stage of wound healing should be noted as this will determine the primary dressing used. A wound swab should be taken if infection is suspected.

Choosing a suitable primary dressing

The ideal primary dressing should maintain wound temperature, retain moisture to facilitate healing, and protect skin surrounding the wound from maceration[16]. Dressings can be divided into three categories: inert, interactive and bioactive. Inert dressings such as gauze and lint should not be used as primary dressings as they do not promote wound healing. Interactive dressings such as gels, films, hydrocolloids and alginates promote wound healing, and the nurse should choose these for primary dressings.

There are currently 371 different dressing materials available on FP10 prescription. Cavity dressings and odour absorbing dressings are not currently available on FP10 prescription to treat the cavity wounds of individuals living in nursing homes. Many nurses in nursing homes obtain much of their information about dressings from representatives of the companies who produce dressings. It is important that nurses are aware that no single dressing is suitable for all types of wounds. Many individuals require different types of dressing as the wound progresses through different stages of healing[17].

The nurse should examine the wound and decide which stage of healing it has reached. The presence of necrotic tissue impedes healing and predisposes wounds to infection. The nurse must examine wounds and decide what she aims to achieve by using a particular type of dressing. Does the wound require debridement? Is exudate a major problem? Is the wound sloughy? The nurse must choose the appropriate dressing for the stage of healing.

Dressings may initially require changing daily but as exudate diminishes they can be left *in situ* for longer periods. As wounds progress the nurse must evaluate the dressing used. If, for example, the wound is no longer exuding heavily then alginate dressing may no longer be appropriate and a hydrocolloid or film dressing may now be the dressing of choice. The nurse has a professional duty when assessing wounds and selecting dressings to document her assessment, choice of dressing, aims, intentions and the outcome of her choice.

Wound cleansing

Antiseptics were developed to kill bacteria but they also kill healthy cells and impede wound healing. Eusol is particularly damaging to wounds, and nurses generally accept that its use cannot be justified[12, 13, 16, 17], although some doctors continue to advocate its use[18]. Providone iodine also inhibits wound healing and can result in increased infection rates[14].

Cetrimide and chlorhexidine also kill healthy cells. The use of hydrogen peroxide can cause similar cellular damage but it can be used just for a short period to remove loose slough and debris from the wound surface[19]. Following irrigation with hydrogen peroxide the wound should be irrigated with warm normal saline so that the hydrogen peroxide is not left in contact with the skin[20]. The use of hydrogen peroxide for a short period to remove wound debris has been shown to expedite wound healing[21]. Normally wounds should be cleaned only if debris is present. Normal saline should be used, and this should be warmed to prevent cooling the wound and delaying healing. Irrigation is preferable to swabbing as swabbing can damage the wound surface and delay healing.

Treatment of venous ulcers

Compression bandaging is now recommended in the treatment of venous ulcers. Compression reduces the superficial venous pressure, improves venous return, reduces oedema and relieves the feelings of aching and heaviness which affect individuals with venous ulceration[22]. Compression therapy should never be used without a thorough assessment to exclude arterial problems. The use of compression therapy in individuals who suffer from arterial problems can cause tissue damage which can lead to the development of gangrene[23]. Community nurses have pioneered the use of Doppler ultrasound which enables individuals with arterial problems to be identified.

Many nurses, fearful of the dangers of compression therapy, continue to bandage venous ulcers with crepe bandages. It has been proved that the use of high compression bandaging dramatically improves healing in venous ulceration[24].

There are four different levels of compression therapy:

(1) light compression is achieved by using crepe or short stretch compression bandages
(2) moderate compression is achieved by the use of paste bandages and an outer bandage
(3) high compression is achieved by the use of compression bandages or compression stockings
(4) extra high compression is achieved by the use of four layer bandaging techniques

Bandages should be applied early in the morning, ideally before the individual is up and about as this is when oedema is least pronounced. Bandages should not be applied so tightly that they impair circulation.

Individuals suffering from venous ulcers should be encouraged to elevate their legs. Using a footstool is not normally sufficient; individuals should be encouraged to lie down on their bed and the legs can be elevated on several pillows so that the legs are higher than the heart. The pillows should be placed lengthwise to avoid calf pressure which could impede venous circulation. This elevation aids venous return and assists healing.

Treatment of ischaemic and mixed aetiology ulcers

The individual's doctor should be asked to refer them to a vascular clinic. Vascular specialists will carry out investigations and determine if it is possible to improve blood supply by the use of drugs or surgery. They may decide that surgical treatment of the wound is required. If this is not indicated they can provide advice on caring for ischaemic wounds and can monitor progress.

Treating the individual using a problem solving approach

The nurse who wishes to provide the best possible care to individuals with wounds must become a 'wound detective'[25]. The nurse has a duty to carry out a comprehensive assessment of the individual who has a wound. Assessment enables the nurse to identify problems which might not have been discovered otherwise. The role of nutrition is critical if wound healing is to occur, and assessment may identify that Mrs Davis has a poor diet because her dentures no longer fit and her mouth is sore. Few nurses would think of calling a dentist when a wound was failing to heal. Mrs Hill may suffer from marked postural oedema and no longer walks about because she cannot get her shoes on. The nurse can organize a referral to an orthotist who can supply shoes to accommodate oedema. Mrs Hill can be encouraged to walk around and walking will improve venous return and reduce oedema.

The nurse should adopt a problem solving approach to wound care and should identify and rectify wherever possible the factors which contributed to the development of the wound. Nurse and patient can work together to identify problems and find solutions which enhance the older person's quality of life.

Preventing recurrence

Many nurses have seen wounds heal only to break down again weeks or months later. Recurrence of chronic wounds can cause individuals to become upset and depressed and nurses can become demoralized asking, 'Why . . . was it my fault? Was it something I did?'.

Using a holistic approach to wound management lessens the chance of wounds breaking down again. Individuals who have not benefited from a holistic approach to wound management are more prone to recurrence. The individual whose iron deficiency anaemia remained undetected and untreated is more at risk than the individual who has received treatment. The individual who has a poor diet lacking in nutrients is more at risk than the individual who is having a healthy diet. The immobile individual is more at risk of recurrence than the individual who has been encouraged and helped to regain mobility.

Individuals with venous ulcers should wear support stockings to aid venous return and prevent recurrence. Support stockings can be obtained by asking the patient's doctor to refer them to the orthotist at the local hospital, the individual is then measured for stockings. There are three different types of compression stockings available:

(1) light support or class 1 stockings are suitable for treating mild varicose veins
(2) medium support or class 2 stockings are suitable for moderately severe varicose veins and can be used to prevent the recurrence of venous ulcers and treat mild oedema
(3) strong support or class 3 stockings are used to treat severe varicose veins and oedema and to prevent recurrence of venous ulceration.

Many individuals are reluctant to wear compression stockings. Women complain that the colours are awful and the stockings look dreadful, but it is now possible to obtain compression stockings in a range of colours and the nurse should ensure that the individual obtains a colour she will be happy wearing. Men usually object to wearing stockings, but thick black compression stockings which look like knee length socks are now available and most men find these acceptable.

Two pairs of stockings are normally supplied. Laundered carefully each pair will last three to six months. Further supplies can be obtained on FP10 prescription from the local pharmacist. The nurse should keep a record of the size and the measurements supplied by the orthotist as the pharmacist will require these.

Compression stockings do not survive normal nursing home laundering. They should be washed by hand in a mild detergent such as washing up liquid. Biological washing powders ruin the carefully selected colour and can irritate delicate newly-healed skin. On no account should elastic stockings be dried in the tumble dryer or put on a hot radiator as they will shrink. They can be dried on a washing line outside or in a warm room. Compression stockings can be difficult to get on. A little talcum powder applied to the leg can help. It is possible to get a special steel frame known as a medi-valet to help put stockings on. The stocking is stretched over the frame and the individual slides the foot into the stocking and pulls the frame up the leg, so applying the stocking.

Problem wounds

Some wounds fail to heal despite the efforts of the nurse. The nurse may lack the expertise to deal with some wounds such as fistulas and ulceration around stoma sites. She may not have access to Doppler ultra sound machinery or she may lack the skills to perform ultra sound measurements. The nurse has a duty to act within her sphere of competence. Admitting that she does not possess specialist skills to care for individuals who have problem wounds is a sign of strength not weakness. The nurse should find out what help is available in her local area, who has the skills and knowledge to help her and how to gain access to that help.

Where to get further information and help

Most health authorities employ stoma care nurses; there is often a hospital and a community based stoma nurse. Health authorities vary in their attitude to nursing homes; some view them as extensions of hospitals and the hospital based stoma care nurse is available to help and advise nurses. In other areas nursing homes are viewed as part of the community and the community based stoma nurse should be contacted. The nurse should check her local health authority policy.

Many health authorities also employ hospital and community based wound care specialists, and the nurse can ask the appropriate one for help and advice. Nurse specialists dealing with diabetes are also employed in hospital and community settings and can be called on for help and advice.

The nurse should find out how to contact these nurse specialists and should note their names and contact numbers. The nurse should not hesitate to contact them; they will welcome enquiries from nurses keen to give the best possible research based care. It is often possible for the nurse working in a nursing home to arrange to spend a day with the nurse specialist, learning about her work and gaining information and skills which can be applied on return to work. Nurse specialists often run or are involved in study days and national Board courses. Getting to know your nurse specialists is a good way of ensuring that you are informed of any relevant study days or national Board courses which you might wish to attend.

Conclusion

Wound care is more than a matter of dressing a wound. The health status of the whole person has contributed to the development of the wound. The nurse who assesses the individual with the wound can identify the factors which contributed to the development of the wound. The nurse can work with the individual, the individual's doctor, nurse specialists and other relevant professionals to help the individual to heal physically and mentally from the effects of the wound.

The nurse has a duty to do the patient no harm. An awareness of the actions of wound cleansing agents and dressings enables the nurse to make informed choices and select appropriate cleansing agents and dressings. The use of compression bandaging is harmful in individuals with arterial disease and of benefit to individuals with venous ulcers. An ability to discover the causes of ulceration enables the nurse to provide appropriate care. The nurse has a duty to remain professionally up to date. Contact with clinical specialists and other professionals can prevent professional isolation and ensure that she is aware of relevant courses and study days.

Useful addresses and telephone numbers

Stoma care nurse

Wound care specialist nurse

Community leg ulcer clinic

References

(1) Callan, M.J., Harper, D.R., Dale, J.J. & Rucklye, C.V. (1987) Chronic ulcer of the leg; clinical history. *British Medical Journal*, 294, 1389–91.
(2) Negus, D. & Friedgood, A. (1983) Effective management of venous ulceration. *British Journal of Surgery*, **70**, 623–7.
(3) Moody, M. (1993) State of the art of wound care: a survey of wound management in nursing homes. Wound care in the community. *Professional Nurse Supplement*, 7–11.
(4) Dale, J. & Gibson, B. (1986) The epidemiology of leg ulcers. *Professional Nurse*, **1** (8), 215–16.

(5) Jones, P.L. & Milman, A. (1990) Wound healing and the aged patient. *Nursing Clinics of North America*, 25, 263–7.

(6) Rosenburg, C.S. (1990) Wound healing in the patient with diabetes mellitus. *Nursing Clinics of North America*, 25, 247–61.

(7) Bryant, R. (1987) Wound repair: a review. *Journal of Enterostomal Therapy*, 14, 262–6.

(8) Papantonia, C.T. (1988) Holistic approach to healing (part 2). *Home Healthcare Nurse*, **6** (6), 31–5.

(9) Dyson, M. et al. (1988) Comparison of the effects of moist and dry conditions on dermal repair. *Journal of Investigative Dermatology*, 12, 434–40.

(10) Lock, P.M. (1979) The effects of wound temperature on mitotic activity at the edge of experimental wounds. Symposium on wound healing (ed. N. Sundell). Espoo, Helsinki, 103–9.

(11) Johnson, A. (1988) The Cleansing Ethic. *Nursing Times*, **84** (6), Community Outlook.

(12) Tatnall, F.M. et al. (1989) Comparative toxicity of antimicrobial agents on transformed human keratinocytes. *Journal of Investigative Dermatology*, 89, 313–17.

(13) Viljanto, J. (1980) Disinfection of surgical wounds without inhibition of normal wound healing. *Archives of Surgery*, 115, 253–6.

(14) Cutting, K. (1944) Factors influencing wound healing. *Nursing Standard*, **8** (5), 33–6.

(15) Moffatt, C. (1993) Assessing leg ulcers. *Practice Nursing*, 21st September – 4th October, 8–10.

(16) Thomas, S. (1990) Wound management and dressings. *The Pharmaceutical Press*, 2, 78.

(17) Turner, T.D. (1985) Which dressing and why. In *Wound Care* (ed. S. Westby). Heinemann Medical Books, London.

(18) Calder, S.J. & Leaper, D.I. (1986) Chronic venous ulcers and the role of dressings in their treatment. *British Medical Journal*, **101** (1), 6–11.

(19) Morrison, M.J. (1989) Wound cleansing, which solution? *The Professional Nurse*, **4** (5), 220–25.

(20) Turner, V.G. (1991) Standardisation of wound care. *Nursing Standard*, **5** (19), 25–8.

(21) Fergusson, A. The best performer. *Nursing Times*, **83** (14), 52–5.

(22) Burnard, K.G. et al. (1988) How effective and long lasting are elastic stockings? In *Phlebology* (eds D. Negus & G. Janter). John Libbey, London.

(23) Callam, M.J., Ruckley, C.V. & Dale, J.J. (1987) Hazards of compression on the treatment of the leg; an estimate from Scottish surgeons. *British Medical Journal*, 295, 1382.

(24) Moffatt, C.J., Franks, J.P., Oldroyd, M. Bosanquet, N. et al. (1992) Community clinics for leg ulcers and impact on healing. *British Medical Journal*, 305, 1389–92.

(25) Eagle, M. (1994) *Wound Care in the Nursing Home*. Nursing Homes Today second national conference, May. Royal College of Nursing, London.

Chapter 7
Continence Promotion

Introduction

Urinary incontinence is a major problem in nursing homes. Research indicates that 60% of older people living in nursing homes suffer from uninvestigated and untreated urinary incontinence. It has a devastating effect on morale, and complications arising from untreated incontinence can cause illness.

Urinary incontinence can cause nursing workload to rise to unmanageable levels, make staff feel useless and increase staff turnover. It can be costly in financial as well as human terms. Nursing time, laundry and incontinence pads for an individual suffering from urinary incontinence total £15 per day or £105 per week. In the average 39 bed nursing home with a 60% incontinence rate £2457 per week is spent solely on dealing with incontinence.

It is possible for nurses to help older people regain continence. Individuals who have done so often take on a new lease of life, take part in activities within the home and go out with friends and relatives once more. Nurses can see that their skills really make a difference and because workload is cut they can spend more time with their patients. The costs of caring for incontinence are greatly reduced.

The causes of incontinence

Continence is a learned skill; we are all born incontinent and as we develop neurological and muscular control of our bodies we learn to become continent. The association of incontinence with infancy and a lack of control is an unfortunate one. As adults we feel that the loss of control associated with incontinence is deeply embarrassing and shameful. Incontinence is one of the last great taboos in our society. In order to maintain continence an individual must be aware of the sensation of bladder fullness, and have the ability to hold on, locate a toilet and adjust clothing and use the toilet. Continence is therefore dependent on a complex system of hormonal, muscular and neurological controls.

The causes of incontinence are equally complex. There is no one single cause and continence cannot be viewed in isolation from other aspects of physical and mental wellbeing. Normal age related changes make it more difficult for older people to remain continent. Urinary incontinence becomes more common with increased age, and research indicates that 15% of elderly people living at home are incontinent[1]. Ageing diminishes the body's reserve capacity and makes it more difficult for older people to maintain homoeostasis. Age related changes to the urinary system combined with an acute illness or the worsening of a chronic disease can tip previously continent older people 'over the edge' and they are more prone to become incontinent when ill than younger people. This is because illness can place a strain not only on the urinary system but on other previously unaffected systems.

Older people living in nursing homes are more disabled and more likely to be acutely ill or suffering from chronic diseases than those living at home[2]. Understanding how ageing affects the urinary system enables nurses to work with older people to help them overcome the difficulties they face in maintaining continence.

How ageing makes it more difficult for people to remain continent

The kidneys become smaller and lighter with age, the weight of the average kidney decreases from 250 g to 200 g between the ages of 20 and 80. The majority of cells lost are in the renal cortex which contains the largest number of functioning glomeruli[1]. It is estimated that the decrease in functioning glomeruli is between 30% and 50% in extreme old age[3]. The surface area of the remaining glomeruli is reduced and there is thickening of the glomerular basement membrane. These structural changes affect the blood flow through the nephrons and decrease the ability to concentrate urine and to maintain PH balance[4]. These changes cause older adults to produce greater volumes of urine. Older people become dehydrated more readily because their kidneys are less able to concentrate urine and preserve fluid.

Arteriosclerosis reduces blood flow to the kidneys from 600 ml per minute at the age of 40 to 300 ml per minute at the age of 80[5]. It has been suggested that this reduction is caused partly by decreased cardiac output and the decreased renal vascular bed[6]. This reduced blood flow causes the kidneys to work less efficiently.

Glomerular filtration rates (GFR) have been shown to decline significantly with age[7]. Older people are more at risk of the toxic effects of drugs which are excreted from the kidney. These include digoxin, cimetidine and cephalosporins. Illness can further lower GFR and can lead to elevated levels of phosphate, uric acid and potassium and lower levels of bicarbonate. These changes mean that older people are more prone to adverse reactions to medication and electrolyte imbalances.

In older people the kidneys are less able to concentrate urine because they become less sensitive to anti-diuretic hormone (ADH). ADH normally concentrates urine and reduces urinary output while we sleep. Many older people have to get up at night to pass urine because they produce large volumes of urine when asleep. Renin activity is diminished with age and this leads to a reduction in aldosterone which can lessen the kidney's ability to reabsorb sodium, potassium and water in the distal tubule.

Older adults are, as a result of these changes, more at risk of electrolyte imbalance. Diuretics increase this risk. One study found that 73% of cases of hyponatraemia in elderly people were caused by diuretic therapy. Older adults are less able to dispose of large fluid loads and they run the risk of cardiac failure resulting from increased blood volume if too much fluid is given too rapidly. Intravenous fluids must be given with particular care because of this risk and nurses must be aware of this risk when encouraging fluids hourly.

The bladder muscle – the detrusor – is smooth muscle which expands and contracts in all directions. The detrusor is primarily under parasympathetic control. Parasympathetic stimulation releases acetylcholine causing detrusor contraction and assisting bladder emptying. Sympathetic control is via the beta-adrenergic receptors which are situated in the body and fundus of the detrusor. Stimulation of these receptors assists in bladder relaxation and filling. The main age related bladder changes are all intrinsically linked. The afferent sensors in the bladder become less sensitive with age. Adults become aware that they need to pass urine when the bladder is 50% full; older adults are not normally aware until their bladders are 90% full. This means that older adults have less time to find a toilet and, when combined with disabilities which impair mobility, this can lead to incontinence. The bladder muscle no longer stretches and contracts as efficiently as before and the amount of fibrotic tissue in the bladder increases, so the bladder is able to hold less urine.

Women continue to produce oestrogen after the menopause but in some cases a lack of oestrogen can effect the urethra and lead to stress incontinence.

Older men have larger prostate glands than younger men, as the prostate gland enlarges with age. This causes problems in a minority of men but if prostatic growth is into the bladder neck (common in prostatic malignancy) this can lead to decreased sphincter control. Benign prostatic enlargement can lead to an increased amount of residual urine because of urethral obstruction. This residual urine, if in excess of 350 ml can cause back flow to the kidneys, renal damage and infection. Older men are much more at risk of urinary tract infections because as they age the prostate produces less prostatic bacteriocide to prevent urinary infections.

The effects of age related changes

Ageing affects the kidneys; they are less efficient at clearing drugs from the body, at maintaining electrolyte balance and at concentrating urine. The bladder can hold less urine than before, is less efficient at emptying, and older people are not aware of a full bladder until it is almost completely full. These changes make it more difficult for people to remain continent as they age.

Many older people are cared for at home before admission to a nursing home. Carers often find urinary incontinence difficult to cope with and encourage older people with severe continence problems to seek nursing home care[7]. Many individuals are admitted to nursing homes from hospital, usually directly after a major illness, accident or because a chronic condition has worsened. Nursing staff and care managers working with older people in hospitals and in the community are more likely to suggest nursing home care when continence problems exist.

Many older people who have continence problems are admitted to nursing homes but few will have benefited from investigations which identify the type of incontinence and the reasons for the problem. Most people are so embarrassed by incontinence that they try to conceal it; they feel that the situation is hopeless[8]. Many nurses feel that they can do little to help older people with continence problems and that incontinence is an inevitable consequence of extreme old age and illness. Fortunately many older people with incontinence can regain continence with the help of skilled nurses.

Types of incontinence

There are six different types of incontinence and the treatment for each is different.

(1) Urge incontinence

This is also referred to as bladder dysreflexia or unstable bladder. It is caused by uncontrolled bladder contractions and leads to leakage of urine. Individuals often leak urine just as they enter the toilet. People with Alzheimer's type dementia, disseminated sclerosis, spinal cord injury or cerebrovascular accidents can develop urge incontinence[9]. It becomes more common as people age even in the absence of disease.

Treatment

Many cases of urge incontinence can be treated by toileting programmes; details are given later in this chapter. Toileting programmes should be used before medication is considered. If they are unsuccessful or only partially successful drug therapy can be considered. Medication acts by 'damping down' bladder contractions. This increases bladder capacity and allows individuals to hold on longer.

The most commonly used drug is oxybutinin but imipramine and propantheline are also used. These drugs are known as anticholinergics. Medication should be given in the smallest possible dose in older people to minimize side effects. Anticholinergics can cause urinary retention. Maintaining a fluid balance chart in the first three weeks of use or if the dosage is increased will alert nurses to this side effect. Other side effects include a dry mouth.

(2) Stress incontinence

This is caused by a urethra which fails to stay closed when intra-abdominal pressure is raised. Small amounts of urine leak if a woman sneezes, coughs, laughs or jumps. It is common in pregnant and post menopausal women and rare in men, usually only occurring after prostatectomy[10].

Treatment

Some women have uterine prolapse and the insertion of a ring pessary can support the uterus, relieving pressure. The insertion of a pessary can restore continence. Ring pessaries can be inserted by GPs with family planning training; they are often coated with oestrogen which further treats stress incontinence. Pessaries are normally changed every 12 months.

Pelvic floor exercises can strengthen the pelvic floor.

Oestrogen treatment enables the urethra to close more efficiently and prevent leakage. Doctors normally prescribe oestrogen cream which is applied vaginally. This is usually given daily initially and then reduced to weekly or monthly as a maintenance dose. Stress incontinence is made worse by coughing; treatment of a chest infection, if one is present, will restore continence. Individuals with chronic chest conditions can be referred to physiotherapists who can teach a method of coughing which does not raise intra-abdominal pressure as much as a normal cough.

Anticholinergic drugs can help some individuals.

Men suffering from stress incontinence following prostatectomy should be referred back to the surgeon who performed the operation for investigation or treatment.

(3) Mixed incontinence

This is a combination of stress and urge incontinence.

Treatment
As indicated above.

(4) Overflow incontinence

This is a condition where the bladder fails to empty properly and the individual leaks small amounts of urine on movement. It can easily be confused with stress incontinence. The commonest cause is faecal impaction. Other causes include enlarged prostate, urethral stricture, Parkinson's disease, diabetes and spinal cord compression[11].

Treatment
The aim of treatment is to enable individuals to empty their bladder completely. Constipation and faecal impaction should be treated if present. Medication that might be causing urinary retention should be reviewed and wherever possible discontinued by medical staff. Nursing measures such as applying a warm flannel to the abdomen and gently tapping the abdomen often help. If these measures are ineffective medical staff should be contacted.

Long term management of chronic urinary retention can include intermittent self catheterisation or an indwelling catheter.

(5) Functional incontinence

This is incontinence which occurs in people with normal bladder function. It is common in people with advanced dementia and head injury.

Treatment
Toileting regimes can restore continence in some individuals with functional incontinence. The continence is entirely dependent on nursing staff toileting and will relapse if nursing staff discontinue toileting.

(6) Transient incontinence

Many older adults or their families report that the incontinence has only just started. Often the patient or relative can tell nurses exactly when and often why incontinence began: 'I was fine until Doctor changed my water tablets'; 'I was managing until my arthritis got so bad I couldn't get to the toilet in time'; 'She was fine until her stroke'. This is known as transient incontinence and older people suffering from it can often be helped to regain continence[12]. The causes of transient incontinence are:

- delirium/confusional state
- infection
- atrophic urethritis/vaginitis
- pharmaceuticals
- psychological – especially depression
- endocrine
- restricted mobility
- stool impaction

Treatment

Confusion often leads to urinary incontinence, but it is often possible to treat the causes of acute confusion and this leads to the individual regaining continence[13].

Drugs can often cause incontinence[14]. Nursing home patients are often prescribed a range of drugs which both inter-react and can cause incontinence[15, 16]. Nurses can inform GPs of any problems and medication can often be changed, discontinued or reduced to a smaller dose[17].

Urinary tract infections often cause older people to become incontinent and many individuals regain contience when treated[18].

The ability to get to the toilet is crucial and research indicates that this is the single most important factor in enabling individuals to regain continence. Individuals may have developed a foot or leg deformity after a cerebrovascular accident, for example, and may require not only physiotherapy but appropriate footwear and possibly callipers to enable them to walk. An individual may have developed leg shortening following repair of hip fracture and may require a raise on a shoe. Nurses can ask GPs to refer older people with mobility problems to orthotists, who can provide specialist footwear, and to physiotherapists.

The ability to adjust and/or remove clothing when in the toilet is essential to maintaining and regaining continence. Nurses can advise older people about clothing which is easy to remove and can show individuals ways of dressing and undressing which take disability into account. The Disabled Living Foundation produce an excellent book which gives guidance on choosing clothes and provides useful dressing techniques for elderly people and people with disabilities[19].

Anxiety and depression make bladder problems worse. Many older people feel depressed when they leave their own homes and enter nursing home care. Nurses can help them by helping them to settle in and by encouraging them to take part in the daily life of the home[20, 21]. Hypothyroidism is sometimes mistaken as depression in older adults and nurses can alert GPs to this possibility.

Faecal impaction is a common cause of urinary incontinence; an impacted bowel can cause outflow obstruction and overflow incontinence. Older men, because of the tendency to prostatic hypertrophy, are particularly at risk of overflow incontinence[22]. Disimpaction resolves the problem and the introduction of a high fibre diet, encouragement of sufficient fluids and mobilization where possible, prevent recurrence without having to resort to laxatives in the majority of cases[23].

How nurses working in nursing homes can promote continence

The nurse working in a nursing home can enable older adults to maintain continence, can investigate and rectify, where possible, the factors leading to transitory incontinence, can promote continence in individuals with established incontinence and can contain incontinence among chronically incontinent patients.

Maintaining continence

A great deal of urinary incontinence within nursing homes and other institutions is caused by nursing practice[24, 25, 26, 27]. A letter published in the nursing press, written by a 22 year old man admitted for investigations of mild urinary incontinence, illustrates this:

> 'When I felt the need to urinate and attempted to find the toilet, an auxiliary nurse escorted me back to my chair and said in a loud voice, "It's OK; you have waterproof pants on . . ." After four days in that place I had "progressed" to wearing adult all-in one diapers . . . and was readily wetting myself instead of using the toilet . . . After seven days I had regressed to being totally dependent on aids . . . I went into hospital a good looking 22 year old with self respect and confidence. I am now totally dependent and rely on baby's underwear.'[28]

The nurse must take a long hard look at working practices within the nursing home if she is to succeed in enabling older adults to maintain continence. One of the greatest dangers of institutionalization is that the abnormal is accepted as normal and that nursing practice actively fosters dependence or 'excess disability'. It is essential that active steps are taken to maintain continence and other life skills if older adults are to enjoy optimal quality of life.

Older adults must be able to identify toilets and should have regular eye tests and glasses, if appropriate, to optimize vision. Treatable eye problems such as cataracts and glaucoma can be detected early and the patient's GP can treat or refer appropriately. The signs on toilets should be large enough to be read by individuals with poor eyesight and pictures of toilets pinned to toilet doors can assist neurologically impaired patients to identify them. There should be sufficient toilets to avoid queuing which can lead to urinary incontinence in individuals with symptoms of urgency. Toilets should be well lit and doorways and toilets large enough to accommodate wheelchairs and walking frames. Raised toilet seats and grab rails can help older people to use the toilet independently or with minimal help.

Older people who can walk to the toilet are less likely to suffer from incontinence than individuals who depend on nurses to take them to the toilet[29, 30, 31]. The goal of skilled nursing care is to prevent or reverse excess disability so that the patient is not prematurely disabled and is functioning to capacity. Nurses can work with older people to prevent them becoming prematurely disabled but many nurses have worked in places where patients have already become prematurely dependent. Nursing can actively foster disability by:

- wheeling patients around rather than encouraging walking 'because its quicker' or 'because it must be such a struggle for poor Mary'
- lifting patients who are able to transfer themselves
- dressing patients who can dress themselves slowly.

In this culture patient ability is rapidly lost and disability, apathy and a sense of powerlessness fostered. A home where older adults are supported, and encouraged to maintain and regain skills, is vital. Older adults must have appropriate footwear, foot and nail care and must not be made to feel slow or clumsy when they move around.

In many nursing homes, as in elderly care wards, beds are routinely covered with plastic sheets and draw sheets whether the patient is continent or not. Nursing staff justify the practice by saying 'just in case', but the message it gives is that urinary incontinence is acceptable and even expected. If continence is to be maintained and incontinence treated, nursing staff must be educated to accept that continence is normal and incontinence abnormal. Incontinence must be reported, investigated and treated. It is possible with a positive attitude to assist older adults to retain independence. An individual who becomes wheelchair bound can often be taught to transfer from chair to toilet. This approach enables older people to retain dignity, independence and a sense of wellbeing for as long as possible.

Investigation and treatment of established incontinence

Established incontinence is incontinence of more than three months' duration[32]. Many older adults enter nursing homes from hospital or from residential homes with established, uninvestigated urinary incontinence. Illness and diseases such as arthritis which impairs mobility[33] and stroke which can impair mobility and cognitive function, can predispose individuals to urinary incontinence[34, 35, 36]. Continence problems are often not documented or acted upon because nursing staff accept incontinence as an inevitable consequence of illness or ageing and do not perceive urinary incontinence as a treatable condition[37]. The extent of urinary incontinence is often masked by 'padding', i.e. giving incontinence pads to patients[38]. This can often cause transient incontinence to be obscured and to progress to established incontinence because continence promotion strategies are not employed early.

It is essential that urinary incontinence is promptly identified on the individual's admission to the nursing home and a detailed assessment carried out either by a GP or a continence adviser. An assessment should include the following:

- history of the incontinence
- onset – sudden or insidious
- precipitant factors
- patient perception
- expectation
- description of symptoms
- obstetric history (if relevant)
- dysparenui
- medical history
- medication
- what makes it worse

A physical examination will enable continence advisers to identify problems and to work with the older person and the nursing staff to promote continence. The examination should be followed by investigations of a simple nature and should include temperature, pulse, blood pressure and respirations. A urinalysis should be carried out and a midstream urine sent to the laboratory for microscopy culture and sensitivity. The patient should be asked to empty their bladder and after this their abdomen should be palpated; it should not be possible to palpate a bladder with a residual urine of less than 100 ml. If the bladder is palpable or palpation is difficult (perhaps because of obesity) then a bladder ultrasound can be carried out. If there are no facilities for ultrasound examination a catheter can be passed and any residual urine measured.

The patient, or in some cases staff caring for the patient, should be asked to maintain a fluid balance chart for one week. This should detail all fluids drunk and should measure where possible all urine output. Episodes of incontinence should be recorded with some indication of the severity of incontinence; this could range from slightly damp to very wet.

BLADDER TRAINING

PROGRAMME

In order to bring your bladder problem under control, you must learn to stretch your bladder. You can do this by trying to hold on as long as possible before passing water. Do not restrict your fluid intake. You should drink no more or less than you normally do.

On the back of this sheet is a bladder chart to help you monitor your progress - fill this in **every time you pass urine normally** and **every time you are wet**.

- ☐ Place a tick in the **shaded** column to the nearest hour when you leak urine, place a tick in the **plain** column when you pass urine normally.

- ☐ When you get the feeling that you want to pass urine **try to hold on for as long as possible.**

- ☐ At first this will be difficult, but as you persevere it will become easier.

- ☐ If you wake up at night with a full bladder it is best to go and empty it straight away, as holding on will only keep you awake.

- ☐ Sitting on a hard seat may help you to hold your water.

- ☐ Your doctor may have prescribed tablets to help you hold your water. Take these regularly as directed.

- ☐ You should aim to gradually reduce the frequency with which you pass urine to 5 or 6 times in 24 hours.

REMEMBER

You are attempting to stretch your bladder. Although you may find this difficult at first, with practice it will get easier. If you persevere, you will be surprised at what you can achieve.

BLADDER CHART

Week commencing:　　　　Name:

Please tick in the **plain** column each time you pass urine

Please tick in the **shaded** column each time you are wet

Special instructions:

	Monday	Tuesday	Wednesday	Thursday	Friday	Saturday	Sunday
Midnight							
1am							
2							
3							
4							
5							
6							
7							
8							
9							
10							
11							
Noon							
1pm							
2							
3							
4							
5							
6							
7							
8							
9							
10							
11							
Totals							

Fig. 7.1 Copy frequency volume chart.

Nursing staff may be asked to fill in a frequency volume chart. This is shown in Fig. 7.1. Each time an individual uses the toilet the left hand column is ticked; every time incontinence occurs the right hand column is ticked. This chart enables nurses to monitor continence. They can easily see if continence is improving and in around two thirds of older people a pattern emerges. This pattern can be used to prevent incontinence; for example if an individual is often wet at 9 AM then a reminder or help to use the toilet at 8:45 AM will often eliminate incontinence. Many older people regain continence using this method. Unfortunately in around a third of older people it is not possible to identify a pattern.

These measures allow the nurse specialist to identify the nature and severity of the problem in the majority of cases, without recourse to urodynamic testing[39]. The nurse specialist has the ability to identify and initiate appropriate treatment for the majority of patients living in nursing homes, and is able to refer more complex cases to the appropriate specialist so that they receive investigation and treatment.

Toileting regimes

Bladder retraining

Bladder retraining encourages older people to retrain their bladders. Many older people get into the habit of going to the toilet very often and the bladder does not get a chance to fill properly. It then becomes smaller; bladder training entails gradually increasing the time between going to the toilet, usually by 10 to 15 minute intervals. The individual eventually uses the toilet at a normal frequency.

Timed Toileting

This is a system where the individual is taken to the toilet at set intervals, usually every two to four hours, and asked to use the toilet. It can help restore continence in individuals following cerebrovascular accident or others suffering from neurological impairment.

Individual toileting schedules

Some older adults may suffer from chronic incontinence and are unable to maintain continence. It is possible in many cases for nursing staff to identify an individual voiding pattern for these individuals and to take them to the toilet at these times to avoid incontinence. Individuals who are regularly toileted must fulfil certain criteria before individualized toileting can be contemplated; they must be able to maintain continence between toileting episodes, have a bladder capacity of at least 200 ml and agree to frequent toileting. Toileting must not be detrimental to their general wellbeing.

These schedules can be maintained by nursing staff without creating an intolerable workload if transient incontinence and established incontinence have been successfully treated in other patients.

A terminally ill individual might prefer to have incontinence contained using a pad or a catheter rather than spend their last days struggling to maintain continence.

Prompted toileting

Many individuals can regain continence if reminded to use the toilet at regular intervals by nursing staff. This is a responsibility which should not be undertaken lightly as any failure to remind an older person can result in incontinence.

Caring for chronically incontinent older adults

It is important that older adults who suffer from urinary incontinence are thoroughly investigated and treatment commenced. Some older adults fail to display a readily identifiable voiding pattern and attempts to establish an individualized voiding schedule are unsuccessful. The nurse specialist can advise nursing staff of the most humane and effective ways to contain incontinence in these individuals, who are usually the most frail of the nursing home population. This normally involves the use of incontinence pads.

Catheters

Indwelling urethral catheters are often seen as the solution to continence problems. We do not know how many older people in UK nursing homes are catheterized. In the US a quarter of all nursing home residents have their incontinence managed with indwelling catheters and it is thought that catheterization is a less expensive option for managing incontinence than pads are. Long term catheterization can cause major problems and older people who have their incontinence managed by this method have shorter life expectancies than those using pads[40] The most common problems are infection, blockage due to incrustation, leakage[41], pain, and urethral trauma.

Catheters are available in a bewildering array of materials, types and sizes. Silicone and hydrogel catheters are most suitable for long term use and normally require changing every twelve weeks. They are available in sizes 12 to 22. It is now recommended that nurses use the smallest possible catheter when catheterizing an individual. It is common practice in many clinical areas to replace a leaking catheter with a catheter a size larger. Individuals can rapidly progress to size 22 catheters but leakage persists.

There are two main reasons why catheters leak. Some individuals have a tendency to encrust catheters rapidly. A change of catheter resolves the problem but it can recur within a few weeks. A range of bladder washouts are manufactured and it is claimed that regular washouts with specific products will prevent blockage. However, bladder washouts are now thought to be of little value in such situations[42] and they can increase the risk of urinary tract infections. In such situations nurses should review the need for catheterization and if possible use alternative methods to manage incontinence.

In many individuals leakage is caused by bladder spasm, and inserting a larger catheter worsens the situation. Constipation and faecal impaction can cause catheters to leak; treatment of constipation can prevent catheter changes.

Catheters now come in two lengths: the shorter one is known as the female catheter and was designed to take account of the fact that women have a shorter urethra than men. Most older women find the shorter length catheter more comfortable and discrete. Men should continue to use longer length catheters.

Catheters are available with different balloon sizes: 5 ml, 10 ml and 30 ml. Large balloons are heavier than smaller balloons and the weight of water pressing on the bladder neck can cause irritation, pain, discomfort and leakage. These problems often resolve if a catheter with a large volume balloon is replaced with a smaller balloon. Nurses should normally only use catheters with 5 to 10 ml balloon sizes.

Male catheterization

It has been traditional that nurses do not insert urethral catheters in male patients. Male catheterization used to be traditionally seen as a doctor's role, arising from the fact that the majority of nurses were once female and the majority of doctors were once male. Now 50% of students entering medical school are women and general nursing is no longer viewed as a female occupation. In response to this changing situation male nurses in many hospitals have been taught to catheterize male patients and hospital policies reflect the fact that male nurses have acquired this skill. Female nurses though are usually not taught the skills of male catheterization. This situation can cause problems in nursing homes where nursing staff are predominantly female[43]. The home has a duty to provide care for the patients who are admitted. In some areas male patients have to wait many hours for catheterization or a catheter change because female nurses lack this skill and are forced to ask busy GPs to visit. The Royal College of Nursing's continence care forum have produced a booklet on the subject of male catheterisation[44]. Nurses can gain such skills and enhance patient care: further details are given at the end of this chapter.

Drainage

In hospital two litre drainage bags are normally used and these are kept on stands which sit by an individual's bed or chair. Leg bags are the preferred option in nursing homes. A bag secured with straps to the leg is more discrete and dignified and will not impede mobility. It is recommended that leg bags are changed every five to seven days. Some older people hate the idea of having a bag which fills with urine being strapped to their leg; even though it is hidden by clothing it can feel uncomfortable and unpleasant. It is now possible to use a valve which closes off the catheter. The bladder stores urine and this is drained off every two to four hours by opening a valve. A drainage bag can be attached for night use if required. Catheter valves are now available on prescription, and some individuals may prefer to use them instead of leg bags.

Faecal incontinence

Few older people suffer from faecal incontinence; it is thought that only 2% of older people have this problem. The number of older people resident in nursing homes who suffer from faecal incontinence is not known. The commonest causes of faecal incontinence are faecal impaction, diarrhoea and neurological diseases. Many drugs commonly prescribed to older people can cause constipation, including analgesics, iron preparations, diuretics, antacids, antidepressants, antihistamines and antiparkinsonian medications. These drugs can cause constipation with overflow. Faecal disimpaction will resolve this situation and restore continence.

Laxative use is common in nursing homes; one study found that 59% of older people in nursing homes were taking laxatives regularly[45]. It is extremely difficult for doctors to calculate and prescribe the correct dosage of laxatives. Irritant laxatives such as senna can cause abdominal pain, cramps and diarrhoea; this can lead to faecal incontinence. Stool softeners can lead to the bowel becoming loaded with soft stool and faecal leakage.

Individuals suffering from constipation benefit from a radical review of medication. If an individual is no longer suffering from iron deficiency anaemia then iron tablets can be discontinued. Nursing measures such as encouraging mobility, elevation of legs whilst sitting and the use of elastic stockings can effectively reduce or eliminate ankle oedema and enable doctors to discontinue diuretics prescribed to control limb oedema. Older people can be encouraged to eat a diet high in fibre which reduces the need for aperients (see Chapter 10).

Nursing practices such as rushing older people when they want to use the toilet or not ensuring that they can open their bowels in privacy can all contribute to constipation. Haemorrhoids and anal fissures can be extremely painful and can cause individuals to be reluctant to defecate; if these problems are suspected they can be easily investigated and treated by the individual's doctor.

Diarrhoea can cause faecal incontinence. Chronic diarrhoea should be investigated and treated. In some cases individuals may be prescribed medication to control diarrhoea and restore normal bowel habit.

Neurological diseases such as cerebrovascular accidents and Alzheimer's type dementia can result in individuals being unaware of when they have opened their bowels. Most people open their bowels after breakfast (or another meal) and if individuals suffering from neurological disease are helped to the toilet after meals and encouraged to open their bowels they can often develop a regular bowel pattern.

Useful address and telephone number

Your local continence adviser

Improving your skills

The ENB 978 course, An introduction to the Promotion of Continence and the Management of Incontinence, is run at a number of centres throughout the UK. The length of the course varies from $5\frac{1}{2}$ days plus clinical placements to 12 days. The course is usually available on a day release basis. The nurse should check when applying that the course is linked to a university and that CATs points are awarded. The course normally has 15 level two CATS points.

A new course ENB A57 is also available. This comprises four modules, is spread over one to three years and carries 60 level two or three credits. Individual modules in continence care are also available at degree level. At the time of writing there is only one UK centre which currently runs diploma and degree level courses. Write for details to R. Addison, Mayday Hospital, London Road, Croydon, Surrey.

Conclusion

The introduction of a continence promotion programme can appear daunting. Nurses who begin such a programme should begin slowly and build on success. The rewards are enormous. Older people freed at last from a sense of shame and worthlessness can regain self respect and independence. Nursing workload is reduced and nursing staff have more time to spend with patients. The promotion of continence is an area where nurses can work with older people to improve quality of life. It is not possible to enable all older people to regain continence, but nurses who gain skills in the management of incontinence can prevent the complications of poorly managed incontinence and can deal with this problem with sensitivity, enabling older people to retain dignity.

Further reading

Articles

These specifically relate to continence promotion in UK nursing homes.

Nazarko, L. (1992) Programmed to succeed. *Nursing the Elderly*, **4** (4) 20–21.
Nazarko, L. (1993) Solving incontinence through assessment. *Nursing Standard*, **8** (6) 25–7.
Nazarko, L. (1993) Preventing constipation. *Elderly Care*, **5** (2) 32–3.
Nazarko, L. (1994) Drugs, continence and elderly people. *Primary Health Care*, **4** (1) 19–22.

Books

Norton, C. (1986) *Nursing for Continence*. Beaconsfield Publishers, Beaconsfield.
Roe, B. & Williams, K. (1994) *Clinical Handbook for Continence Care*. Scutari, Harrow.

Sources of further information

Continence Care Forum, Royal College of Nursing, 20 Cavendish Square, London W1M 0AB. Tel. 0171 409 3333.
Continence Foundation, The Basement, 2 Doughty Street, London WC1 2PH. Tel. 0171 404 6875. The Continence Foundation produces a range of information including a continence resource pack. Individual copies are available free.
Incontinence Information Hotline (open Monday to Friday 2pm to 7pm) Tel. 0191 213 0050.

References

(1) Hellstrom, L., Ekeland, P., Milsom, I. & Mellstrom, D. (1990) The prevalence of urinary incontinence and the use of incontinence aids in 85 year old men and women. *Age & Ageing*, **19** (6), 383–9.

(2) Ouslander, J.G., Moriskita, L., Blanstein, J. *et al.* (1987) Clinical functional and psychosocial characteristics of an incontinent nursing home population. *Journal of Gerontology*, **42** (6), 631–7.

(3) Lindeman, R.D. (1981) Kidney. In *CRC Handbook of Aging* (ed. E.J. Mason), 175–91. CRC Press, Florida.

(4) Bonomi, V. & Vangelista, A. (1988) Structural and functional changes in the elderly. *Clinical Nephrology*, 61, 74–81.

(5) Roberts, A. (1989) Systems of life no 169, senior systems no 34. The ageing urinary system. *Nursing Times*, **85** (10), 59–61.

(6) Rowe, J.W. (1988) Renal system. In *Geriatric Medicine* (2nd edn) (eds J.W. Rowe & R.W. Besdine), 231–45. Little, Brown and Co., Boston.

(7) Ouslander, J.G., Zarit, S.H., Orr, N.K. & Muira, S.A. (1990) Incontinence among elderly community dwelling dementia patients; characteristics, management and impact on care givers. *Journal of the American Medical Association*, 38, 440–45.

(8) Wyman, J.F., Harkness, S.H., Choi, S.C., Taylor, J.R. & Fantyl, A. (1987) Psychological impact of urinary incontinence in women. *Obstetrics and Gynaecology*, **70** (3), 378–81.

(9) Wells, T.J., Brink, C.A. & Diokono, A.C. (1987) Urinary incontinence in women – clinical findings. *Journal of the American Geriatric Society*, **35**, 933–9.

(10) Delancy, J.O. (1990) Functional anatomy of the female urinary tract and pelvic floor. Proceedings of Ciba Foundation symposium 151, 57–76.

(11) Brocklehurst, J. (1984) Ageing, bladder function and incontinence. In *Urology in the Elderly*. (ed. J.C. Brocklehurst), Churchill Livingstone, Edinburgh.

(12) Resnick, N.M. (1984) Urinary incontinence in the elderly. *Medical Grand Rounds*, 3, 281–90.

(13) Resnick, N.M. & Paillard, M. (1984) Natural history of noscominal incontinence. Proceedings of the 14th annual meeting, ICS, Innsbruck, 471–2.

(14) Blandy, J.P. (1989) *Lecture Notes on Urology* (4th edn). Blackwell Science, Oxford.

(15) Hatton, P. (1990) Primum non nocere – an analysis of drugs prescribed to elderly patients in private nursing homes registered with Harrogate Health Authority. *Care of the Elderly*, **2** (4), 166–8.

(16) Primrose, W.R., Capell, A.E. & Simpson, G.E. (1987) Prescribing patterns in registered nursing homes and long stay wards. *Age and Ageing*, 16, 25–8.

(17) Nazarko, L. (1994) Drugs, continence and elderly people. *Primary Health Care*, **4** (1), 19–22.

(18) Diokono, A.C. (1988) The causes of urinary incontinence. *Topics in Geriatric Rehabilitation*, 3, 13–20.

(19) All Dressed Up... (1994) Disabled Living Foundation, 380–384 Harrow Road, London W9 2HU.

(20) Sutherland, S. (1971) Emotional aspects of incontinence in the elderly. *Modern Geriatrics*, May, 270–4.

(21) Wells, T. (1984) Social and psychological implications of incontinence. In *Urology in the Elderly* (ed. J.C. Brocklehurst), 107–26. Churchill-Livingstone, Edinburgh.

(22) Brown, R.B. (1982) Clinical Urology Illustrated, 73–5. Adis Press, Sydney, Australia.

(23) Nazarko, L. (1993) Preventing constipation. *Elderly Care*, **5** (2), 32–4.

(24) Willington, F.L. (1969) Problems of urinary incontinence in the aged. *Gerontologica Clinica*, 2, 330–56.

(25) Calder, M. (1976) The Nursing of Incontinence. In *Incontinence in the Elderly* (ed. F.L. Wellington) 202–9. Academic Press, London.

(26) Miller, A. (1985) A study of the dependency of elderly patients in wards using different methods of nursing care. *Age and Ageing*, 14, 132–8.

(27) Miller, A. (1985) Nurse/patient dependency – is it iatrogenic? *Journal of Advanced Nursing*, 10, 63–9.

(28) Cullodine, S. (1987) Urinary incontinence – a lesson for nurses. (Letter in *Nursing Times*), 83, 14.

(29) Ouslander, J.G., Kane, R.L., Abrass, I.B. (1982) Urinary incontinence in elderly nursing home patients. *Journal of the American Medical Association*, **348** (10), 1194–8.

(30) Ouslander, J.G., Morishita, L., Blaustein, J., Orzeck, S., Dunn, S. & Sayre, J. (1987) Clinical functional and psychosocial characteristics of an incontinent nursing home population. *Journal of Gerontology*, 42, 631–7.

(31) Ouslander, J.G., Ulman, G.C., Urman, H.N. & Ruberstein, L.Z. (1987) Incontinence among nursing home patients; clinical and functional correlates. *Journal of the American Geriatric Society*, 35, 324–30.

(32) Resnick, N.M. (1984) Urinary incontinence in the elderly. *Medical Grand Rounds*, 3, 281–90.

(33) Yarell, J. & St Leger, A. (1979) The prevalence, severity and factors associated with urinary incontinence in a random sample of the elderly. *Age & Ageing*, 8, 81–5.

(34) Borrie, M., Campbell, A. & Carodoc, D.T. (1986) Urinary incontinence after stroke: a prospective study. *Age and Ageing*, 15, 177–81.

(35) Brocklehurst, J., Andrews, K. & Richards, B. (1985) Incidence and correlates of incontinence in stroke patients. *Journal of American Geriatric Society*, **33** (8), 540–2.

(36) Rottkamp, B. (1985) A holistic approach to identifying factors associated with an altered pattern of urinary elimination in stroke patients. *Journal of Neurosurgical Nursing*, 17 (1), 37–44.

(37) Palmer, M.H., McCormick, K.A. & Langford, A. (1989) Do nurses consistently document incontinence? *Journal of Gerontological Nursing*, **15** (12), 11–16.

(38) Stater, P. & Libow, L.S. (1985) Obscuring urinary incontinence: diapering the elderly. *Journal of the American Geriatric Society*, 33, 842–6.

(39) Dennis, P.J., Rohner, T.J., Hu, W.T., Igou, J.F., Yu, L.C. & Kaltreider,

D.L. (1991) Simple urodynamic evaluation of incontinent elderly female nursing home patients: descriptive analysis. *Urology*, 32 (2), 173–9.

(40) Platt, R., Polk, B.F., Murdock, B. & Rosner, B. (1983) Reduction of mortality associated with noscominal urinary tract infection. *New England Journal of Medicine*, 307, 637–42.

(41) Roe, B.H. & Brocklehurst, J.C. (1987) Study of patients with indwelling catheters. *Journal of Advanced Nursing*, 12, 713–18.

(42) Roe, B.H. (1993) Catheter associated urinary tract infection. *Journal of Clinical Nursing*, **2** (4), 197–204.

(43) Seccombe, I., Ball, J. & Patch, A. (1993) *The price of commitment, nurse's pay, careers and prospects.* Report 251, 34, 49–52, 65–66. Institute of Manpower Studies, Brighton.

(44) Guidelines on Male Catheterisation (1994) Royal College of Nursing Continence Care Forum. RCN, London.

(45) Primrose, W.R., Capell, A.E. & Simpson, G.E. (1987) Prescribing patterns observed in registered nursing homes and long stay geriatric wards. *Age and Ageing*, 16, 25.

Chapter 8
Preventing Pressure Sores

Introduction

The incidence of pressure sores in UK nursing homes is not known. Research indicates that the incidence of pressure sores in UK hospitals is 15%, and in NHS elderly care units varies from 4% to 34%. The majority of people in NHS hospitals who have pressure sores have developed them in hospital[1]. Older people who live in nursing homes are particularly at risk of developing pressure sores. Some nurses feel that it is inevitable that some frail and terminally ill older people will develop pressure sores in the nursing home. Almost all pressure sores are preventable. The goal of skilled professional care is to assess risk and rectify, wherever possible, factors which predispose to pressure sores. Care should be planned to prevent the development of pressure sores.

Pressure sores – why nursing home patients are at risk

A pressure sore is an area of cellular damage. It is caused by unrelieved pressure on the skin or shearing forces. Shearing forces can occur when an individual is lifted or moved. Blood supply is interrupted and tissue death occurs. Anyone, of any age will develop pressure sores if the skin is subject to unrelieved pressure, but it is recognized that certain groups of people are at greater risk.

Older people are at particular risk of developing pressure sores for a number of reasons. Chronic illness and its physical effects make an individual more likely to develop pressure sores. Immobility increases the risk because immobile people are not able to relieve pressure by moving and are dependent on others to do this for them. Individuals who are not lucid or who are drowsy, often because of the effects of medication, are less aware of pressure on skin. They are less likely to complain of discomfort and are often dependent on nursing staff to relieve pressure. Individuals who have sensory loss, perhaps as the result of diabetic induced peripheral neuropathy, or other neurological problems are often unaware of pressure and discomfort and are dependent on nursing staff to relieve pressure. Individuals with cardiac and arterial problems suffer from compromised circulation. Blood flow to tissues is reduced and damage can occur more readily than in individuals with a healthy circulation.

Nutrition is a very important factor in the development of pressure sores[2]. Obesity can predispose an individual to pressure sores as adipose tissue has a poorer blood supply than normal tissue. Very thin older people are at extremely high risk of developing pressure sores. Some older people have skin which is more prone to damage than others. Individuals on long term steroid therapy and others who have thin papery skin are more prone to develop tissue damage.

Urinary incontinence can make an individual more likely to develop a pressure sore[3]. Urine can cause dermatitis, maceration and excoriation of the skin. Any skin damage increases the risk of pressure sores.

Older people who live in nursing homes are among the most disabled

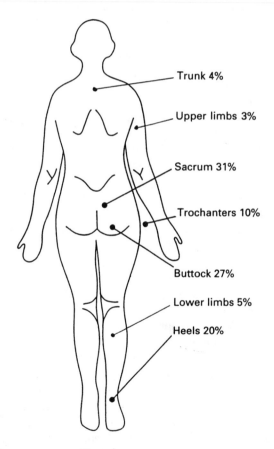

Fig. 8.1 The common position of pressure sores.

of their generation. They are more likely to suffer from chronic illness, more likely to have impaired levels of consciousness, more likely to suffer from neurological disease and more likely to be admitted in a malnourished state[4]. Urinary incontinence is a major problem in nursing homes. The older person admitted to a nursing home is extremely vulnerable and at high risk of developing pressure sores. The goal of skilled professional nursing care is to prevent pressure sores developing and to heal any pressure sores present on admission.

Assessing and reducing risks

It is essential that the home uses a risk assessment scale to determine the level of risk for each individual. There are a number of risk assessment scales. Each scale scores risk factors and the scores indicate to the nurse the individual's risk of developing a pressure sore. The Norton score assesses five risk factors[5]. The Waterlow score includes other factors such as age, nutritional status, skin type and diseases including those which affect circulation[6]. Nursing staff at the home should decide which scoring system will be used. The score should be determined on admission, but it must be stressed that scoring is an ongoing process and should be carried out whenever there is a major change in an individual's condition. Routine scoring also helps detect individuals whose risk factors have slowly changed.

In many areas nurses focus solely on using aids to relieve pressure when an individual is identified as being at risk of developing a pressure sore. Holistic care involves the nurse working with the individual and other professionals to rectify any possible factors which increase the risk of pressure sores.

Mobility is a key factor in the development of pressure sores. Ensuring that the individual has suitable shoes and aids, organizing physiotherapy, and helping the individual to exercise and regain mobility, reduce the risk of pressure sores.

Nutrition is an important factor. Ensuring that the individual is supplied with a healthy balanced diet with sufficient nutrients, calories and protein reduces the risk of tissue breakdown.

Treatment of any cardiovascular disease and gentle exercise improves circulation and reduces risk.

Use nursing measures to promote sleep, and have realistic expectations about the sleep requirements of older people. Encouraging exercise and leisure activities will make older people feel more alert. It is unlikely that such individuals will require hypnotics to help them sleep; their days will be full and active and they should sleep well. The risk of the individual developing pressure sores is further reduced.

Poorly managed urinary incontinence predisposes an older person to tissue breakdown. Many nurses feel an indwelling urinary catheter reduces the risk of an individual developing pressure sores and is an essential part of treatment if the individual is incontinent and has a pressure sore. Many individuals are admitted to nursing homes with urinary catheters *in situ* and some nurses fear that if they remove the catheter they will increase the risk of an individual developing a pressure sore. Urinary catheterization increases the risk of infection and is associated with increased mortality rates. Urinary catheters should only be used if clinically indicated (see Chapter 7).

The goal of skilled nursing care should be to promote continence wherever possible. If it is not possible for the individual to regain continence the aim of nursing care should be to contain incontinence and prevent skin damage. The skin should be washed after each episode of incontinence, using a gentle soap which does not dry the skin. If the skin is becoming very dry, plain water should be used. A barrier cream may be required. This should be applied lightly as using too much cream can interfere with the ability of incontinence pads to absorb urine. Incontinence pads should be chosen with care. A good quality pad which contains a gel draws urine away from the skin and locks it into the pad. Some older people are so distressed by the fact that they have a urinary catheter that they do not wish to get better. Many can, with the help of skilled professional nursing, recover their zest for life.

> Margaret Mitchell was admitted to a nursing home following repair of a fractured femur. She was immobile, had a urinary catheter *in situ*, was suffering from a large deep pressure sore to her sacrum and had lost all will to live. She was malnourished, in pain and curled into a foetal position. Her glasses had been lost and she could see little without them. Analgesia was given, the wound swabbed and redressed and admission procedures completed.
>
> Margaret was at her lowest ebb and felt that she had come to the nursing home to die. The admitting nurse worked with Margaret to identify her needs and ensure that these were met. Margaret's catheter which made her feel 'dirty and smelly' was removed and she regained continence using continence promotion strategies as detailed in Chapter 7. She regained mobility when provided with suitable shoes, a frame, glasses and physiotherapy (see Chapter 11). Nutritional needs were met, her wound was dressed and pressure relieving devices were used. Margaret regained not only mobility and continence but also her self respect and zest for life.

Pressure relieving aids

Individuals at low risk of developing pressure sores – those who do not suffer from chronic illness, who are not malnourished, who have no sensory loss and who are not incontinent – are still at risk of developing pressure sores, if their skin is subject to unrelieved pressure for more than a few hours. Elderly people who are at risk of developing pressure sores may suffer from tissue damage even if their position is changed every two hours.

The areas of the body most at risk of ischaemic damage are the sacrum, heels, buttocks and greater trochanters. Almost half of all pressure sores develop on the sacrum and almost 20% develop on the heels[7]. The aim of pressure relieving aids is to relieve and redistribute pressure to avoid tissue damage. The ideal mattress should be capable of redistributing pressure, should be impermeable and easily cleaned, should allow the skin to breathe, ensure patient comfort, enable nursing staff to provide care without restriction and be competitively priced and affordable. Unfortunately the ideal mattress does not exist. A range of pressure relieving overlays and mattresses exist. Foam overlays, ripple mattresses and low air loss beds are all available. Assessment of risk enables the nurse to choose the appropriate pressure relieving overlay or mattress to prevent the development of, or treat existing, pressure sores.

Working with the individual to reduce risk factors enables the use of less expensive foam overlays on the majority of beds. These are indicated for use on the beds of individuals with Waterlow scores of between 10 and 15. Individuals who have a Waterlow score of 15 to 20 should be nursed on overlays which alternate pressure. Ripple mattresses are often used for individuals in this category. A number of ripple mattresses are available; price and specifications vary. The nurse should ask for details of each product prior to purchase. Some ripple mattresses are suitable for people at greater risk than others; for example, one product is suitable for individuals with a Waterlow score of 20 whilst another is only suitable for individuals with a score of 15.

Guarantees vary; some manufacturers only offer a three month guarantee on the mattress and six months on the motor whilst others offer a full twelve month guarantee on both motor and mattress. It is important that the nurse is able to have defective mattresses repaired quickly. Older people entering nursing home care are now more dependent than ever before. Nursing staff may find they require more ripple mattresses if they are to prevent pressure sores. The temptation is to buy as many as possible within the budget but this should be resisted and nurses should ask suppliers to supply a mattress on loan for a period of time. Most suppliers will send a representative to visit the home. The representative will provide technical details and copies of relevant research reports and papers relating to the product and its use in preventing or treating pressure sores. Nursing staff will be shown how to use the product, which is loaned for approximately four weeks. Nursing staff can then compare and evaluate products before purchase. A product which appears less expensive but is unreliable or less effective may well be the most expensive in the long term. Ripple mattresses cost from £300 to £500 each. The budget conscious nurse should always ask for a discount if more than one is being purchased.

Individuals who are at extremely high risk of developing pressure sores or who have already developed pressure sores may require specialist mattresses or beds. Low air loss beds and mattresses are used in some nursing homes. Low air loss mattresses are extremely expensive to purchase at around £3000. They can be hired from manufacturers on a weekly basis at a cost of approximately £60 per week. They are extremely effective at preventing pressure sores and facilitate healing. Some homes only receive £296 per week for providing care to extremely dependent older people so may find the cost of hiring a low air loss bed prohibitive.

If an older person is admitted to the home with an existing pressure sore and the use of a low air loss mattress is clinically indicated then social services should be informed of this. The nurse can then negotiate with the care manager about the provision of the mattress. In some areas social services departments hire and pay the costs directly; in others the home is paid a higher fee which covers this cost. Details of such arrangements should be included in the individual contract issued by social services and countersigned by the nurse and care manager.

If an individual deteriorates and requires specialist equipment the care manager should be contacted to organize an emergency care review so that such matters can be settled. Individuals responsible for paying their own fees or with preserved rights status are not the responsibility of social services. It may be possible to borrow a bed from the stores department of the community trust – see Chapter 11 for details.

Individuals at risk of developing pressure sores are equally at risk of sustaining tissue damage when seated in a chair. The nurse should ensure that a range of foam, gel and ripple cushions are available and are used appropriately to prevent tissue damage when the individual is sitting in a chair.

A range of aids are available to protect heels. Heel protectors and boots are designed to reduce pressure and reduce shearing forces. Heel blocks, shaped like bricks with a U shape cut in them, support the ankles and hold the heels clear of the bed. A ring cushion (now recognized as an inadequate means of relieving sacral pressure) can be placed under each foot so that the heel is suspended and pressure is relieved when the individual is in bed.

Aids are intended to serve as a supplement to and not a substitute for nursing care, which should include relieving pressure two hourly.

Assessing wounds

Pressure sores are preventable in the vast majority of cases if individuals receive high quality individualized patient care which meets their needs. Caring for individuals who are at extremely high risk of developing pressure sores, and preventing their occurrence, is a mark of high quality professional care. The incidence of pressure sores is an important indicator of care. Many individuals are admitted to nursing homes with pressure sores acquired either in hospital or in the community. It is not always possible to determine either the presence of or the extent of a pressure sore during an assessment visit.

All individuals admitted to a nursing home should have their risk assessed on admission. This is important as the individual's condition (and risk factors) may have changed since the initial assessment. Individuals who have pressure sores should have a full assessment. This should include the site of the wound and its size. A record of the wound size and depth should be made. A grid can be used to trace the wound and the depth can be measured with a probe. Some homes provide a Polaroid camera so that a photograph can be taken.

There are two widely used methods of classifying pressure sores. One classifies wounds in five categories[8], whilst another uses four categories[9]. Senior nursing staff within the home should determine which classification system they will use, and the classification should be recorded.

These are the details of the classification scheme used by Torrance:

Stage 1   Reddening is present. Light finger pressure causes the skin to whiten, referred to as 'blanching hyperaemia'. The whitening indicates that capillary circulation is intact and undamaged.

Stage 2   Reddening remains when light finger pressure is applied. This is referred to as 'non blanching hyperaemia' and indicates that capillary circulation is damaged. The skin may be broken.

Stage 3   The skin is ulcerated and subcutaneous tissue is ulcerated.

Stage 4   The ulcer extends into subcutaneous fat. Underlying muscle is inflamed and swollen.

Stage 5   The ulcer extends into muscle or bone.

A wound assessment chart (Fig. 8.2) can be used to provide a baseline measure of the wound. This can be updated at each dressing change.

Treatment of pressure sores

The principles of wound care are given in Chapter 6. Individuals who have pressure sores are at risk of developing infection; details of infection control strategies are outlined in Chapter 5.

The care of people who have cavity wounds presents a particular challenge to nurses working in nursing homes. Cavity wounds form as a

Name:	Date: ....
Position of wound	**Type of wound**
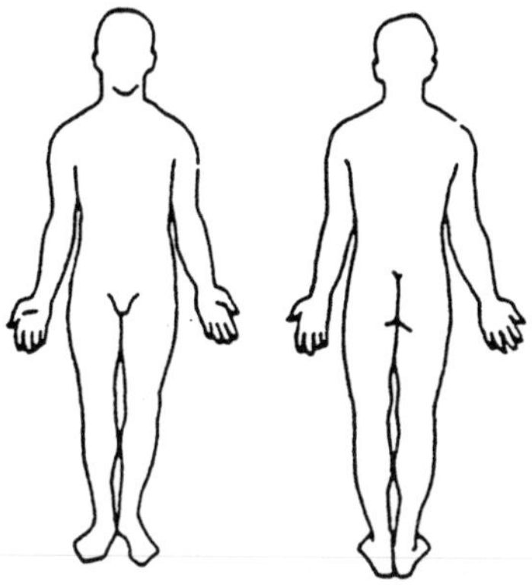	Associated problems

Wound appearance: *Other comments:*

Necrotic: ☐   Deep: ☐

Clinically infected: ☐   Shallow: ☐

Sloughy: ☐   Offensive: ☐

Granulating: ☐   Heavy exudate: ☐

Epithelializing: ☐   Size in cm .....

Suggested plan:

Fig. 8.2 Wound care chart.

result of deep tissue loss and they heal by second intention. Granulation tissue from the base of the wound progressively fills the wound as healing takes place. It is important that the appropriate dressing is chosen: the dressing material should prevent sinus formation, facilitate the removal of necrotic tissue and absorb exudate, whilst maintaining optimum conditions for wound healing by maintaining a warm moist atmosphere.

Dressings should be easy to remove in order to avoid damaging granulation tissue. The primary dressings of choice for deep cavity wounds with a high exudate are alginate rope, hydrogel, hydrocolloid pastes and polyurethane foam.

The primary dressings of choice for moderately exuding cavity wounds include alginate dressings, hydrocolloid pastes and hydrogel[10]. Alginate rope is not available on FP10 prescription. Nurses wishing to pack cavity wounds can tease apart the fibres on alginate dressings and lightly pack the wound with this material. Hydrogel is available in three sizes within the NHS (8, 15 and 25 g) but only one size is available on FP10 prescription: the 15 g, which does not contain sufficient hydrogel to pack a large deep cavity wound and the nurse may have to use two or three packs at each dressing change. Hydrocolloid pastes are not available on FP10 prescription.

Malodorous wounds

Deep extensive pressure sores, especially those affecting the buttocks and sacrum, can fill with foul smelling necrotic material. Pressure sores in the sacral region are prone to contamination and colonization by anaerobic bacteria. Anaerobic bacteria produce nauseating odours which can permeate not only the individual's room but large areas of the home. This is extremely distressing to the individual and is offensive to other residents and visitors. Treatment of the underlying infection with an appropriate systemic or topical antibiotic often fails to reduce odour for some days.

The use of dressings containing activated charcoal cloth effectively contains odours. Four dressings are produced specifically to absorb odour in such circumstances, but none are available on FP10 prescription. This may be because doctors and other clinicians who do not work in the nursing home environment are unaware of the range of care provided within nursing homes. One wound care guide states that nursing homes offer 'intermittent nursing care' and care for 'less severe wounds'[11].

Hydrogel can be used to reduce or eliminate the odour of malodorous infected wounds. It can only be used whilst the individual is under medical supervision and the patient must be having systemic antibiotic therapy. A *non occlusive* secondary dressing must be used and dressings must be changed daily[12].

Documentation

Assessment of individuals who have acquired or who are at risk of developing pressure sores should be ongoing. The nursing care plan should indicate this continuing process and should record changes in risk factors. The nurse should document findings, intention, action and outcome when delivering care. Documentation safeguards the nurse from accusations of failing to provide appropriate care. We live in a changing world and individuals and their relatives are more likely to consider legal action if they feel care has been inadequate. In such situations, if care is not documented there is no proof that it has been provided. Many nurses give care but fail to document that care. Some mean to write it up later but get interrupted and never get around to documenting it.

Staff education

The nurse has a professional duty to remain clinically up to date and to provide care which is research based. The nurse working in a nursing home works with care assistants or nursing auxiliaries who have not benefited from professional training. Most care assistants are unaware of the factors which contribute to the development of pressure sores. They may be unaware of the importance of relieving pressure two hourly and of the damage friction can cause to skin. They may have been taught to give reddened skin a good rub; such action can further damage a compromised circulation and contribute to tissue damage. The nurse has a duty to explain the principles of treatment to care assistants who work in the home. Staff who understand the reasons why care is carried out in a certain way are able to work with the nurse to ensure continuity of care.

Conclusion

Pressure sores cause pain and suffering, and can lead to infection and even death. Individuals who develop pressure sores, especially extensive cavity wounds, require high levels of skilled nursing care. It is important that care is holistic and patient centred and meets the individual's needs. The vast majority of pressure sores are preventable. The goal of skilled professional care should be to act to prevent the development of pressure sores rather than react to their occurrence. Preventative strategies include using pressure relieving aids to redistribute pressure.

References

(1) McSweeney, P. (1993) *A study of the implementation of pressure area care in North Essex*. Colchester/North Essex Health Authority.
(2) Agarwel, N. *et al.* (1985) The role of nutrition in the management of pressure sores. In *Chronic Ulcers of the Skin* (ed. B.K. Lee) p. 133–45.
(3) Exton-Smith, N. (1987) The patient's not for turning. *Nursing Times*, **83** (42) 42–4.
(4) Hepple, J., Bowler, I. & Bowman, C.E. (1989) A survey of private nursing homes in Weston Super Mare. *Age & Ageing*, 18, 61–3.
(5) Norton, D. *et al.* (1962) *An investigation of geriatric nursing problems in hospital*. National Corporation for the Care of Old People, London.
(6) Waterlow, J. (1988) The Waterlow card for prevention and management

of pressure sores: towards a pocket policy. *Care, Science and Practice,* **6** (1) 8–12.

(7) Dealy, C. (1991) The size of the pressure sore problem. *Journal of Advanced Nursing,* 16, 663–70.

(8) Torrance, C. (1983) *Pressure Sores: Aetiology Treatment and Prevention.* Croom Helm, Beckenham.

(9) Ward, A.B. *Prescribers' Journal,* **30** (6) 253–64.

(10) Thomas, S. (1990) *Wound Management and Dressings,* p. 86–7. Pharmaceutical Press, London.

(11) *The Wound Programme.* (1992) Centre for Medical Education, University of Dundee, Scotland.

(12) Williams, C. (1988) Intrasite Gel: a hydrogel dressing. *British Journal of Nursing,* **3** (16) 843–6.

Chapter 9
Patient Safety

Introduction

Many older people are admitted to nursing homes with a history of falls. Older people are particularly at risk of severely injuring themselves as a result of falls because many suffer from osteoporosis. Some older people, as a result of illness, are less able to see or detect hazards which can lead to accidents. Relatives and friends of older people are often anxious that the individual will be protected from accidents stating, 'You won't let her fall will you?'.

The nurse has a duty of care and this duty requires the nurse to protect individuals from hazards within the home. It is not possible though to provide a totally safe environment. All actions involve risk. The duty of the nurse is to take reasonable care to avoid risk, to work with older people to assess the risks involved in daily living, and to work towards minimizing risks whilst enabling the older person to live life according to their wishes.

Protecting individuals from hazards

The nurse must comply with legislation enacted to protect individuals from hazard. The Control of Substances Hazardous to Health (COSHH) regulations require staff within homes to ensure that chemicals are stored safely and do not present a hazard to individuals. Domestic supplies such as bleach, toilet cleaners and other cleaning chemicals are covered by COSHH legislation. These should be stored in locked cupboards. In many homes domestic staff use trolleys to transport the equipment and chemicals which they use when cleaning the home; in others boxes are used. Trolleys and boxes containing chemicals should not be left unattended in patient areas.

Many homes have treatment rooms. Medication is normally stored in the drug trolley which should be locked at all times and fastened to the wall, and additional supplies are usually stored in a locked cupboard. It is good practice to store medication such as creams and lotions for external use in a separate cupboard and such medications are often

111

stored in cupboards under the sink. Treatment rooms usually contain a fridge which is also used to store medication. In many homes there are no locks on either the fridge or under-sink cupboards; in this case the treatment room should be locked to prevent access. The nurse has a duty of care under COSHH regulations to protect the older people in her care from preventable hazards. The home should have written policies on such issues.

The home should have a written health and safety policy which should be available to all staff. This should stress the duty that all staff have to protect patients and staff from preventable accidents. Staff should ensure that items are not left lying around on the floor which could cause someone to trip over and fall. Domestic staff should be supplied with large movable notices which enable them to warn of wet floors. It is important that all staff, including domestic, catering, laundry and maintenance staff, are aware of the need to report hazards and prevent accidents. Each member of the team should be aware of the important role they play in maintaining the safest possible environment.

Faulty equipment can cause accidents. The home should employ maintenance staff to maintain equipment in working order and to repair faulty equipment. The nurse should emphasize that all staff must report faulty equipment immediately. A wheelchair with faulty brakes can cause an individual to fall. Any faulty equipment should be labelled faulty and not used until repairs have been carried out. Adequate lighting is also important; older people can easily slip if they are forced to move around in dark or poorly lit areas.

Nurses within homes are generally responsible for ensuring that maintenance staff are informed of faulty equipment and that repairs have been carried out. It is good practice to use a maintenance book. Details of the date and the nature of work required should be entered by staff and the date and time repairs were carried out entered by the maintenance staff. Recording hazards in a book as soon as possible after noticing them helps prevent accidents by ensuring that repairs are not forgotten and that matters are attended to quickly.

Why accidents occur

Most accidents in nursing homes are falls. Individuals can fall over whilst walking, fall out of chairs, fall off toilets or commodes, or fall out of bed. The consequences of a fall range from fracture requiring surgery to minor injuries. Whilst it is impossible to provide a totally safe environment and eliminate falls, nurses should not accept them as inevitable.

The nurse has a professional responsibility to attempt to discover the reason for the fall. If an older person starts falling the nurse should ask why.

Many older people who develop *chest infections* become unsteady and at risk of falling before developing signs such as pyrexia, dyspnea and cough. A referral to the individual's doctor and treatment of any acute illness such as chest infection restores health and lessens the risk of falls.

Postural hypotension can be idiopathic or caused by anti-hypertensive drugs. The individual suffering from postural hypotension stands up, becomes dizzy and falls. The nurse should ask older people, 'What happened? Why did you fall?'. If the nurse suspects postural hypotension, lying and standing blood pressures should be measured. The older person's doctor can be asked to reassess any prescribed medication which can cause postural hypotension. If the hypotension is idiopathic in origin support stockings can be worn. These prevent rapid pooling of blood in the legs when standing and can alleviate postural hypotension. The nurse should explain why the individual feels dizzy when standing up and advise that the individual gets up slowly.

Anaemia results in a reduction of haemoglobin and can cause older people to become dizzy. If an older person is falling the possibility of anaemia should be considered. The older person's doctor can arrange for a full blood count and any anaemia detected can be treated.

Cardiac disease can impair arterial circulation. This can result in older people becoming dizzy and liable to fall. If an older person has symptoms of cardiac disease, treatment by their doctor can reduce the risk of falls.

Neurological impairment, especially following strokes, can increase the risk of falling. Many individuals suffer from gait problems after strokes. Referral to an orthotist will ensure that special shoes are supplied to correct talipes and callipers are supplied if required. Ensuring that older people who suffer from gait problems after strokes are supplied with aids and shoes to correct deformity, reduces the risk of falling[1].

Medication can cause falls. Older people are more likely to suffer from adverse effects of medication. Ageing affects renal and hepatic systems so drugs take longer to clear the system.

Night sedation is commonly prescribed to older people living in nursing homes; research demonstrates that 33% to 45% of nursing home residents regularly take night sedation[2]. Night sedation can cause daytime drowsiness and can make older people more likely to fall. Sedatives and antidepressants also increase the risk of falling[3]. They are frequently used; one survey revealed that between 35% and 45% of older people in nursing homes were prescribed psychotropic drugs[4]. A policy of reviewing prescribed medication with an individual's doctor will reduce the risk of falls. Further details of medication review are given in Chapter 4.

Muscle weakness increases the risk of falling[5] and encouraging older people to take part in exercise programmes to build muscle strength increases mobility and independence and reduces the risk of falling. Details of exercise sessions are given in Chapter 12.

Unsuitable footwear can cause falls. Older people suffering from oedema are often unable to wear their shoes so they wear slippers. If foot oedema is marked, individuals often buy larger slippers which are wide enough to accommodate the oedema but flop off easily. Some nurses cut slippers at the front to accommodate oedema. Such practices increase the risk of falls. It is possible to obtain special shoes designed to accommodate oedema.

Repair of fractured femur using 'pinning and plating' often results in the ligaments in the affected leg becoming stretched. Many older people have one leg longer than the other after such surgery, and the difference in leg length can be as much as 2 in (5 cm). This causes imbalance and increases the risk of falling. Shoes with a raise to equalize leg length will enable the older person to walk more easily.

Specialist footwear can be obtained from the orthotist, who is usually based in the surgical appliance department at the local hospital. The individual's doctor refers to the orthotist who normally visits the home, assesses the problem and orders suitable footwear to correct deformity. Specialist footwear is provided free of charge to older people but the costs of the footwear are charged to the doctor's budget.

Environmental factors contribute to falls. Poor lighting, slippery floors and other hazards can lead to falls. Nurses should do everything possible to ensure that the environment is as safe as possible.

Inadequate seating can lead to falls. Many nursing homes provide comfortable chairs but do not provide special chairs for profoundly disabled older people. Some older people are so profoundly disabled that they cannot sit safely in armchairs designed for domestic use. Individuals who have suffered from strokes may require special chairs which provide support.

Several companies specialize in providing chairs in which profoundly disabled people can safely and comfortably sit. These chairs must be purchased and can be made specially for the individual. They can include features such as a head and/or neck rest, a seat which is sloped backwards slightly making it less likely that the individual will fall forwards and out of the seat, lumbar supports, and soft wedges to ensure that the individual does not become twisted and uncomfortable. They can have specially designed footrests which attach to the chairs with Velcro to increase patient safety and comfort.

The company representative normally visits the home, assesses the individual and suggests how safe and comfortable seating can be provided. The chair is then made to measure. The costs of such specialist chairs vary from company to company and can range from £500 to £950 for the same specification chair. It is worth getting a few quotes from different companies. Chairs can be purchased by the home or the individual. Chairs purchased by the home for an individual are exempt from Value Added Tax (VAT) if a VAT exemption form is completed. The company supplying the chair should be able to supply the relevant form. Chairs purchased by the home can be altered to accommodate other profoundly disabled people at a later date. These adaptions can be carried out by the company for less than £100 in most cases.

Preventing accidents

The nurse who can identify the cause of an accident can use a problem solving approach to prevent the accident recurring. Ensuring that illness is treated can prevent accidents recurring. An awareness of the side effects of medication and alerting the individual's doctor to the problem can prevent further accidents. Ensuring that older people have suitable footwear will reduce the risk of accidents. Encouraging older people to exercise and regain strength will reduce the possibility of accidents. Working with all the staff in the home to ensure that health and safety and COSHH policies are enforced reduces the risk of accident.

The use of preventive measures, assessing the reasons for falling and using a problem solving approach can protect individuals at risk of falling and reduce the incidence of falls.

The consequences of falls

Falls can cause serious injury to older people. Fractures can occur necessitating hospital treatment. In other cases older people can be shaken and upset and reluctant to walk, and can become immobile. Immobility can lead to rapid decline in health and loss of function[6].

Falls can cause nurses to feel guilty and blame themselves for the fall occurring. In this situation the nurse should attempt to ascertain the reason for the fall and wherever possible use a problem solving approach to prevent further falls. Discussing these feelings with a senior member of the nursing staff may help to put the situation in perspective.

Relatives and friends may feel angry and seek to blame nursing staff for failing to prevent falls. It is all too easy in such situations for nurses to over-react and become so concerned with preventing falls that the quality of life, not only of the older person who has fallen but of all the nursing home residents, becomes affected. Nurses in such situations might discourage older people from walking, people who do not walk cannot, after all, fall over. Such action can have a major impact on an older person's health. Discouraging mobility can lead to a loss of muscle strength and loss of independence; continence status can be affected and constipation can occur; depression can result and send the older person on a downward spiral.

Restraint

Nurses use restraint to prevent older people hurting themselves[7]. There are several types of restraint: physical, chemical and cultural.

The physical restraints most commonly used are cotsides, Buxton chairs, tables and lockers. The use of cotsides on beds of all nursing home residents, to prevent falls, was considered good practice in this country less than ten years ago. Research has shown, however, that cotsides can increase the risk of patient injury[8]. Older people who wish to get out of bed may climb over cotsides, which present a greater hazard than the risk of the individual falling out of bed. There have been reports of older people breaking arms and legs when limbs became trapped in cotsides. Restraint can even lead to death[9]. Buxton chairs are rarely used in nursing homes but are still in widespread use in NHS elderly care hospitals.

Chemical restraint is the use of drugs such as night sedation and psychotropic medication which cause drowsiness. Chemical restraint by affecting the level of consciousness can predispose older people to falls.

Cultural factors and nursing practice can restrain older people. Individuals who cannot walk without a frame can have the frame left out of reach. This action can be deliberate or simply thoughtless, but an older person who is dependent on a frame and attempts to walk without it is at risk of falling.

The legal position

Older people living in nursing homes have the same legal rights as people living in their own homes. It is illegal to restrain someone without their consent. It is also illegal to restrain an individual on someone else's instructions. Nurses, though, have a duty of care. If a nurse saw an individual in the kitchen about to burn herself on a gas ring the nurse would be failing in her duty of care if she did not intervene to attempt to prevent an accident.

The issue of restraint raises ethical dilemmas for the nurse. How can the duty of care be reconciled with enabling the older person to make meaningful decisions about their day to day life? Guidance on the issue of restraint has been issued by the Royal College of Nursing, and the issues are explored in detail[10].

Restraint should only be considered as a last resort after all other avenues and alternatives have been exhausted. Its use should be noted on the care plan and reviewed on a frequent basis. The individual should agree to the restraint used, e.g. the use of a cotside. This consent should be documented in the care plan, as consent is required if the use of restraint is to remain within the law. Confused individuals should be asked for their consent during a lucid period and relatives should be aware and agree that this is the individual's wish. The use of restraint should be a rare and not a routine occurrence within the nursing home.

The rights of older people

Life is full of risks and all of us calculate risks and decide if the benefits of taking the risk outweigh the risks entailed[11]. Older people have just as much right to make those decisions as we have. An older person who has poor balance has the right to continue to walk but runs the risk of falling. An older person who is blind has the right to walk freely through the home. The individual can expect that the nurse will exercise a duty of care and ensure that staff do not carelessly leave the home littered with obstacles. The individual takes the risk of tripping over another resident's handbag or bumping into furniture which residents have moved. Details of risk assessment and the decisions which older people make should be recorded in the care plan.

The care plan should reflect the hopes and aspirations of the individual and not the desire of the nurse or relative to maintain safety at all costs. Sometimes the price of maintaining safety is to remove the very things which make life worth living for an older person. They may well prefer to continue with a pleasurable activity even though it carries an element of risk which the nurse and the individual's family are uneasy about.

> Mrs Edith Ellington, an 89 year old widow, was a keen bird-watcher. A birdtable was placed in the garden at the nursing home and Mrs Ellington fed the birds each day. She enjoyed sitting in a chair in the garden at dusk watching the birds. Mrs Ellington became increasingly unsteady on her feet but declined offers of assistance to help her to her chair in the garden. 'It's the only chance I have to get away from you all – my last bit of peace and independence,' she would tell nursing staff. Mrs Ellington stumbled in the garden and fractured her wrist. As soon as she was able, she returned to the garden. Mrs Ellington's family were horrified and felt that nursing staff should wheel Mrs Ellington out to the garden in a wheelchair and remain with her until she wished to return. This suggestion represented a fate worse than death to Mrs Ellington, who had every right to make her own decisions and to live her life as she saw fit. Nursing staff supported Mrs Ellington in her decision, and her family, though anxious, came to accept her rights.

Assessing risks

It is very easy to overestimate the risks older people face within nursing homes. A problem solving approach will help eliminate or reduce many factors which lead older people to fall.

The aim of nursing home care is to support older people and enable them to live as normal a life as possible in an environment where they receive help and support. The nursing home should be as much like home as possible. Yet it is so easy for homes caring for older people to become institutions where routine takes over from providing holistic, patient-centred care. The need to protect individuals, to avoid being blamed for falls, the desire to keep powerful people such as relatives and registration officers happy, can lead us to lose sight of the individual we are caring for. The great danger of institutions is that the abnormal becomes accepted as normal and we lose sight of how older people living at home lead their lives.

Older people live at home for decades and rarely fall out of bed. As soon as the older person enters a hospital or nursing home where nursing practice is defensive and reactive, they are perceived as being at risk of falling. Nurses are led to believe that if an older person is left in bed without cotsides *in situ* and falls, the nurses will be judged to be negligent.

The goal of skilled nursing care should be to focus on older people's remaining abilities and to work with them to minimize the effects of any disability. The nurse who adopts this philosophy cannot justify the introduction of blanket rules which affect the dignity and freedom of older people. It is essential to assess the actual risks individuals face and to weigh up the risks against the losses the individual faces by avoiding risks.

Gains and losses

Older people who do not walk are not at risk of falling over. They face enormous risks though if they become immobile. Muscle strength is rapidly lost. The ability to perform basic activities of daily living is lost, sometimes forever. The individual loses the ability to move freely around the home, to go to the toilet, to chat with friends. Loss of ability to carry out the basic activities of daily living can lead an individual to feel powerless, dependent and vulnerable. Life can no longer seem worth living and the individual can lose self respect[12]. An individual who is encouraged to walk, and to regain muscle strength and functional ability may well fall over many times. But they may well feel that the gains made by regaining mobility and function outweigh the possible risks of falling.

In 1994 33 older people have been reported to have injured themselves whilst bathing in nursing homes and NHS elderly care units. Some older people turned on hot water and scalded themselves, and others slipped. Some health authorities, nursing home managers and nursing home inspectors have reacted by recommending policies which would prevent older people from bathing alone.

Nurses have a duty of care to ensure that older people who are at serious risk should be supervised whilst bathing. A confused older person who is at great risk of injury should be supervised and the nurse who fails to provide supervision could be guilty of negligence. It is important though, to ensure that the lives of the $168\,000$[13] older people who live in nursing homes are not impoverished because a few people are at risk. Older people have as much right to bathe in privacy as any other citizen. They have the right to be assisted into a bath (if they require help), to be provided with a means of summoning help (such as a call bell), and the right to be assisted to get out of the bath safely.

Introducing and implementing blanket policies which affect the freedom of all older people cannot be justified by caring, thinking nurses who seek to care for older people as individuals. If an older person is not at risk or the risk of injury is very low, the loss of individual freedom and privacy far outweighs the small gain in terms of safety. The goal of skilled professional nursing care must be to work with older people to determine the level of risk and a strategy which enables them to take risks as we do ourselves.

Working with older people to determine risks

Many older people at risk of falling are quite prepared to accept that risk. Nurses are often more worried about an older person falling over than the individual concerned is. Nurses worry that they will be considered negligent or incompetent if an older person repeatedly falls. They worry about the risk of serious injury. They worry about the disapproval of relatives who may complain that they did not take proper care of the individual. They worry that the matron/manager of the home will blame them if falls occur. They worry that registration officers will feel that they are not providing adequate care and supervision.

An atmosphere where nurses are supported, guided and helped is essential if older people are to retain control of their own lives. Nurses have a duty to assess risk and provide an environment where older people can make decisions about how they lead their lives in an environment which is as safe as possible. The decision to take a risk, though, is ultimately the individual's decision and not the nurse's.

Working with relatives, managers and registration

Relatives care deeply for the older person who is being cared for in the nursing home. In many cases they have provided support and physical care for many years prior to the individual being admitted to the nursing home. Sometimes relatives feel guilty that they could not continue to provide care for their loved one. Relatives who have done everything humanely possible to care for an older person can sometimes resent the fact that nursing staff appear to be providing care so effortlessly when they struggled to provide care and were unable to cope. It is important that nurses acknowledge the contribution that relatives have made in caring for their loved one. Often relatives feel 'locked out' and excluded from continuing to care.

Caring relatives can be a great asset and should be encouraged to work with nursing staff to provide the highest possible care. They can take part in treatment programmes under the guidance of professional staff and can work with nursing staff to provide continuity of care. Some relatives lead busy lives and have a family of their own to care for but wish to remain involved, perhaps by taking their loved one out on trips. This should be encouraged.

Relatives who have a good relationship with nursing staff, who are aware of the hopes and aspirations of the older person and how nursing staff are working to fulfil these, will be the greatest assets nurses could hope to have. Relatives who are aware of the home's risk assessment and risk taking policies and know that the aims of these policies are to enable older people to make real choices about their lives, will support nurses.

Nursing home managers and matrons wish to provide the best possible care and will work with nurses to formulate policies which deliver quality care. Registration officers can become concerned if accident rates appear high. They may fear that accident rates indicate inadequate staffing levels or that older people are not being given assistance when required. It is important that registration officers are aware of the home's policies on assessment of risk and risk management strategies. Registration officers are keen to avoid the dangers of homes becoming institutions where all individuality is swamped beneath blanket policies.

The importance of documentation

Every nursing home should have a policy on risk assessment. This should include investigating and working with other professionals to eliminate factors which can cause falls and accidents.

A policy on the rights of older people to take risks and a policy on risk management should be written. These need not be lengthy documents; an A4 page on each will suffice. These policies should be explained to older people, their families and registration officers who may wish to have copies.

It is important to document risk assessment in the care plan. This documentation should include factors identified, nursing aims, intentions, actions, outcome and evaluation. Documentation ensures that all staff are aware of the plan of treatment and it protects the nurse from allegations of incompetence or negligence. Such allegations are rare but it is good practice to document all care. Evaluation of care is an important aspect of risk assessment and management. Such evaluation enables nurses to check if their initial assessments of risk were correct. The individual who regained mobility may now be at less risk of falling and may be able to have greater levels of independence than before.

Recording accidents

The nurse has a duty to record all accidents. The policy for documenting accidents varies from area to area and indeed new registration officers working for the same health authority may recommend different forms of documentation. Some health authorities recommend the use of a bound book whilst others favour loose-leafed forms which are filed in an individual's case notes and in an accident folder.

Nurses can learn important lessons from accidents and can often take action to prevent accidents recurring. It is good practice for two or more nurses to review on a regular basis all accidents which occurred in the home. The author undertakes accident reviews monthly.

There can be an increase of accidents at certain times of the day, perhaps when nursing staff are particularly busy. An accident review gives nurses an opportunity to discuss the reasons for accidents occurring at particular times, and to discuss ways of reorganizing nursing workload so that more nursing staff are available to assist and supervise older people during these periods. Nurses should discuss and comment on any action to be taken as the result of each individual accident review, and these comments should be noted in the accident book and initialled by all nurses who participated. If any of the actions involve a proposed change in an individual's care this should be discussed with the individual and noted in the care plan.

Conclusion

Nurses who are aware of the reasons why older people fall can assess individuals who are at risk of falling. Identifying the cause of falls enables the nurse to work with other professionals to eliminate risk factors in many cases. This reduces the risk of accidents.

The nurse must exercise a duty of care and act at all times to maintain the safety of individuals living in the nursing home. Older people living in nursing homes have the same rights as other citizens and it is illegal to restrain individuals without their consent. Individuals have the right to take risks and to make meaningful decisions about how they lead their lives. The nurse has a responsibility to work with older people, their families and other professionals to ensure that the risks of harm are reduced.

The nursing home should have a written policy on assessment of individuals who are at risk of injuring themselves and a policy on risk management. Nurses must document their actions and intentions and the outcome of care. Nurses who work to reduce and eliminate risk factors, wherever possible, and work with older people to enable them to lead a fulfilling life, are able to enhance an older person's quality of life.

References

(1) Meldrum, D. & Finn, A.M. (1993) An investigation of balance function in elderly subjects who have and have not fallen. *Physiotherapy*, **79** (12) 839–42.

(2) Hatton, P. (1990) Primum non nocere – an analysis of drugs prescribed to elderly patients in private nursing homes registered with Harrogate Health Authority. *Care of the Elderly*, **2** (4) 166–8.

(3) Edwards, L.H. (1993) Commentary on antidepressants and falls among elderly people in long term care. *Aone's Leadership Perspective*, **1** (1) 21.

(4) Humphreys, H.I. & Kassab, J. (1986) An investigation into private sector nursing and residential home care for the elderly in North Wales. *Journal of the Royal College of General Practitioners*, 36, 500–3.

(5) Simpson, J.M. (1993) Elderly people at risk of falling; the role of muscle weakness. *Physiotherapy*, **79** (12) 831–5.

(6) Miller, M. (1975) Iatrogenic and neurogenic effects of prolonged immobilisation of the ill elderly. *Journal of the American Geriatric Society*, 23, 360–9.

(7) Ramprogus, V. & Gibson, J. (1991) Assessing restraints. *Nursing Times*, **87** (26) 45–7.

(8) Lund, C. & Sheafer, M. (1985) Is your patient about to fall? *Journal of Gerontological Nursing*, **11** (4) 34–41.

(9) Dube, A. & Mitchell, E. (1985) Accidental strangulation from restraint. *Journal of the American Medical Association*, 256, 2725–6.

(10) *Focus on Restraint* (1988) RCN guidelines on the use of restraint in the care of elderly people. Scutari Press, Harrow.

(11) *The right to take risks.* (1993) Counsel and Care, London.

(12) Nystrom, A.E.M. & Segesten, K.M. (1994) On sources of powerlessness in nursing home life. *Journal of Advanced Nursing*, **19** (1) 124–33.

(13) Laing, W.D. & Buisson, A. (1994) Market Survey, Laing & Buisson.

Chapter 10
Nutrition

Introduction

A balanced diet is essential to maintain health. A healthy diet should contain a wide range of food and provide the optimum balance of carbohydrate, protein, fat, vitamins and trace elements. It should provide sufficient calories to meet the individual's metabolic needs. A diet too high in calories can lead to obesity, can place an additional strain on an older person's heart and can worsen any existing cardiac disease. Obesity can place an additional strain on arthritic joints and make it more difficult for an older person to walk. Hypertension is often worsened by obesity, and wounds heal more slowly in obese individuals.

A diet too low in calories can lead to weight loss. Initially the body metabolizes fat stores but when these are exhausted muscle tissue is broken down. Thin malnourished individuals are at greater risk of infection and pressure sores, and wound healing is impaired. Older people who appear to be of average build can lack vitamins and minerals. Older people are especially at risk of suffering from deficiencies of iron, vitamins B_1, B_{12}, C and D. People over the age of 80 are twice as likely to suffer from malnutrition as other adults[1].

Individuals living in nursing homes are usually extremely disabled and often suffer from a number of chronic diseases. Physical problems may make it difficult for them to eat a normal diet. Most nursing homes are small units; the average nursing home has 39 beds. Many homes employ chefs and cooks who provide excellent food but have little specialist knowledge of the dietary needs of acutely or chronically ill older people. Nursing homes, unlike hospitals, do not employ dieticians.

Nurses have a greater knowledge of the dietary needs of individuals living in nursing homes than any other members of staff employed within the home. It is the nurse's responsibility to ensure that individuals living in the home are given suitable diets. The nurse needs to be aware of the range of special diets individuals may require. A knowledge of conditions which can cause eating difficulties can enable the nurse to offer a suitable diet. Older people are individuals and their dietary needs can vary greatly. A diet that is adequate for one individual may be grossly inadequate for another.

Nutritional needs of older people

The Department of Health has produced two reports which provide comprehensive guidance on the specific intakes of calories, carbohydrate, protein, fat, vitamins and trace elements required. These are expressed in terms of dietary reference values (DRVs) and are statistical estimates of the average needs of older people[2, 3]. People normally become less active as they age, and as levels of activity lessen people require fewer calories. Older people normally require fewer than younger more active people. Older people, though, continue to require at least the same levels of vitamins and minerals as younger people.

Individuals living in nursing homes can have very different dietary requirements. Providing all individuals with the same diet will lead to some individuals becoming malnourished, resulting in poor health. One research study carried out in an NHS long stay unit investigated the reasons why some individuals lost weight whilst receiving what appeared to be an adequate diet. This study revealed that the individuals concerned ate all the food provided and were not suffering from malabsorption or metabolic disorders, but they were all slow or clumsy eaters or were dependent on nursing staff to feed them. All had difficulty in communication and were unable to tell nursing staff that they were hungry. None of them had access to snacks. The reason for their weight loss was that they were simply not getting enough food to meet their requirements. This has been termed 'institutional starvation'[4]. Individuals living in nursing homes are particularly at risk of malnutrition for the following reasons:

- some residents will have difficulty feeding themselves and will be dependent on nursing staff for feeding
- many will be receiving medication which may impair appetite or interfere with the absorption of nutrients
- individuals are dependent on the home to provide meals
- some individuals do not have relatives or friends to provide the snacks with which all patients in all care settings traditionally supplement their diets
- most individuals are suffering from physical or mental disabilities which resulted in their coming to live in a nursing home.

How illness affects the ability to eat a balanced diet

Illness can make it difficult for older people to eat. Loss of the use of a limb, neurological problems, arthritis or weakness can cause older people to experience problems cutting up food and transferring it from plate to mouth. Illness can lead to problems with chewing and swallowing. Understanding the problems older people face and using a problem solving approach can help them enjoy a balanced diet.

Parkinson's disease can cause intention tremor, resulting in food slipping off the fork or spoon which can be very embarrassing to older people. Prescribed antiparkinsonian medication given an hour before meals often reduces intention tremor and enables individuals to enjoy a meal in company without the fear of dropping food. The individual's doctor is often able to adjust the times prescribed medication is given if informed of eating problems.

Individuals with neurological problems as a result of conditions such as strokes, multiple sclerosis or motor neurone disease can have problems with fine muscle control. Food may slide across the plate when the individual is attempting to eat, or the plate may slip or move. The use of plate guards can prevent food sliding off plates, and special anti-slip mats can be placed under plates and bowls to prevent them moving.

Individuals who are hemiplegic experience great difficulty in cutting up food and may have to rely on nursing staff to do this. Providing cutlery specially designed for people who can only use one hand can enable individuals to retain independence. This cutlery has a knife edge on one side and fork prongs on the other. A plate guard should be provided, at least until the individual has become used to cutting and spearing food one handedly.

Arthritic individuals can find it difficult to grip cutlery. Providing special cutlery with hand grips can enable older people to retain independence. Arthritic individuals can sometimes find commercially produced cutlery with grips too heavy to use. Foam insulation designed to keep pipes from freezing can be bought from DIY shops. This is sold by the metre and costs less than a pound. A sleeve of this foam, designed for 15 mm pipes, fits neatly around normal cutlery, providing very light but easy to grip cutlery. The foam slips off easily so that the cutlery can be washed. When the foam becomes grubby it is thrown away.

Pottery cups and mugs full of tea can be too heavy for arthritic and frail older people. Nurses often offer lightweight plastic feeding cups in these circumstances. Melamine cups and mugs are lightweight and look just like ordinary cups, so are a more dignified alternative in many cases. These can be obtained from supermarkets and hardware shops. They are normally used for picnics, and budget conscious nurses will stock up on them in autumn when shops reduce prices.

Some older people have extremely poor eyesight or are partially sighted. Individuals who have suffered from visual loss because of glaucoma tend to lose peripheral vision. Food at the edges of the plate may remain uneaten because it cannot be seen. Using a large plate and placing all the food in the centre of it can enable some partially sighted people to see their meal.

Individuals who suffer from macular degeneration and peripheral neuropathy can distinguish red, black and yellow more readily than other colours. Mashed potato, fish and cauliflower presented on a white plate may be invisible to some partially sighted individuals. Black, red or yellow plates provide a contrast and enable individuals to see the food on the plate. Such plates can be difficult to obtain and extremely expensive, but are available in melamine in shops and hardware stores, where they are sold for picnics.

Individuals can develop hemienopia after strokes and may only be able to see half of the food on the plate. The individual should be encouraged to look around and should be shown the uneaten portion of food. If this is ineffective, placing all the food on the half of the plate the individual can see will usually help.

Older people often complain that 'food doesn't have any taste any more'. Taste buds atrophy with age and older people often use more sugar and salt than before to add taste to food. Yet it is often assumed that older people prefer bland food. Many nursing homes offer mild cheddar when extra mature may well taste like mild to an older person. A bland diet can be boring and unappetising. Nurses should encourage the home's chef to offer tasty alternatives to the traditional nursing home diet. Chilli con carne, pizza or jellied eels may tempt jaded appetites, and variety is the spice of life.

The amount of saliva produced declines with age. Older people may find some food too dry to eat easily. The nurse can ensure that water and drinks are provided with the meal so that individuals can wash their food down.

Oesophageal peristalsis declines with age and some older people can find swallowing difficult. Advising such individuals to take smaller mouthfuls, to chew food thoroughly and to wash food down with a drink, will help.

Strokes can affect fine muscle control of the tongue, jaw and lips. This can make chewing difficult and dentures can slip whilst eating. Fastidious older people can be mortified when they develop these problems and may prefer to go hungry rather than 'show themselves up' in public. This situation requires careful handling. Food always tastes better when eaten in company but if an individual is embarrassed by eating difficulties meals can be served in the person's room. It is important to emphasize to the person that this is at their request and not because nursing staff or patients find their eating difficulties offensive.

Many people regain fine muscle control of the lips, jaw and tongue spontaneously after a stroke, but speech therapists can teach people exercises which help speed up this process. As control improves the individual should be encouraged to join other patients and enjoy a meal in company. Eating alone is rarely as pleasurable as eating with others.

The vast majority of older people wear dentures. Many older people have had their dentures for many years and some dentures no longer fit as well as they once did. Poorly fitting dentures reduce an older person's ability to eat a wide range of foods and can cause gums to become painful[5]. Many older people benefit from having new dentures; others can benefit from having dentures adjusted or relined to ensure a more comfortable fit. Very frail individuals can have temporary soft liners fitted to their dentures to relieve pain and discomfort. Information on obtaining dental services is given in Chapter 11.

How medication affects appetite and nutritional needs

Older people are more likely to suffer from long standing illness than younger people are[6] and many take prescribed medication. This can predispose an older person to malnutrition.

Many older people who live in nursing homes are prescribed sedatives and night sedation[7]. Sedatives can reduce the level of alertness and can lead an older person to lose interest in eating. Nursing measures can often promote sleep and eliminate the need for night sedation; details are given in Chapter 9. Nursing practice can dramatically reduce the use of sedatives; details are given in chapter 3.

Anorexia and nausea are common side effects of many prescribed drugs. Nurses should check how much individuals are eating and if appetite is poor the nurse should consider the possibility of drug induced anorexia or nausea. The older person's doctor can be asked to review medication. Some medication can predispose an older person to vitamin or mineral deficiencies; phenytoin may inhibit the absorption of folic acid and lead to megoblastic anaemia; anti-inflammatory drugs may cause gastro-intestinal bleeding and lead to iron deficiency anaemia[8].

Individuals with special dietary needs

Older people who have wounds, pressure sores or have undergone a recent operation require additional protein, vitamins and calories to enable healing to take place[9]. Active people require larger helpings of food than the inactive. Some older people are very active and can have very high calorie requirements. Older people suffering from dementia who walk around the home constantly may be unable to tell nursing staff that they are hungry, and if they are not offered sufficient food to meet their requirements they can rapidly lose weight.

Some older people are unable to chew food as a result of illness; other older people suffering from end stage dementia tend to spit out meat and lumpy food. Some can manage to swallow a soft diet but in many cases food must be puréed. It is easy to underfeed individuals who are having a puréed diet as liquid added makes portions appear larger than they actually are. Meat and vegetables should be puréed separately and not mixed together. The older person can then choose to eat preferred foods and can leave food which is not liked. If food is mixed together it appears unappetising and a person has no choice but to eat it all or refuse it all. Individual puréed foods can melt into each other on a plate and look unappetising. Pottery or stainless steel serving dishes with three compartments, designed for serving vegetables, can be used to keep meat, potato and vegetable purées separate.

Special diets

The incidence of diabetes rises with age. The pancreas becomes less efficient at producing insulin as adults age. Some older people are thought to become less sensitive to the effects of insulin as a result of age.

Many older people suffer from maturity onset diabetes. This is usually controlled by either diet or diet and oral hypoglaecemic drugs.

The treatment of diabetes has changed dramatically. Twenty years ago diabetics were advised to weigh food and the aim of diabetic treatment was to avoid blood sugars which were higher than 4–6 m.mols, the normal range in non diabetics. This was replaced by a more liberal approach to diet and people with diabetes were taught to measure units of 10 g of carbohydrate, known as portions. A typical diabetic diet might consist of three portions of carbohydrate for breakfast, a one portion snack mid morning, a three portion lunch, a one portion tea, a three portion dinner, and a one portion bedtime snack. People with diabetes were advised to eat foods high in fat but low in carbohydrate, such as cheese and eggs, if the diet failed to satisfy appetite.

Now people with diabetes, of normal weight, are advised to eat a diet high in fibre and low in fat, with sufficient carbohydrate allowed to satisfy hunger. Older people who are overweight and diabetic are usually advised to lose weight. This, together with avoiding sugar and sweet foods, often controls diabetes.

Normally the aim in diabetic management is to maintain blood sugar at levels which avoid the risk of hypoglycaemia and avoid the long term risks of hyperglycaemia. Hyperglycaemia can, in the long term, lead to renal failure, peripheral neuropathy and diabetic retinopathy. These changes take decades to occur.

Older people with maturity onset diabetes who are living in nursing homes are usually in their 80s and 90s and their diabetes is usually of recent onset. Most physicians specializing in diabetes do not consider older people who develop maturity onset diabetes to be at serious risk of the long term effects of hyperglycaemia. They tend to adopt a more liberal approach to diabetic control in such patients. It is generally agreed that older people who are noninsulin dependent and are not suffering any ill effects from their diabetes, such as drowsiness or thirst, can safely maintain blood sugars of 10 m.mol. Maintaining blood sugars which are higher than normal is thought to be preferable to exposing older people to the risks of hypoglycaemia.

Oral hypoglaecemic drugs act by stimulating the islets of langerhans in the pancreas to produce more insulin and are prescribed if diabetes is not controlled by diet. Advice on diabetic diets can be obtained from community based dieticians who can provide dietary advice for nurses and patients.

Insulin dependent diabetes is less common in older people. Community based diabetic nurse specialists will visit older people with diabetes and provide advice on treatment and diet.

Vegetarians

Increasing numbers of people have become vegetarian. Some people eliminate meat from their diet but continue to eat fish, eggs and dairy products. Other people consume no animal products and are known as vegans. Particular care must be taken to ensure that a vegan diet is varied and balanced and supplies trace elements and nutrients. Vegans can be at risk of iron deficiency anaemia but a diet rich in fruit (especially apricots), cereals, nuts, beans and lentils avoids deficiency. Green leafy vegetables (especially broccoli) reduce the risk of folate deficiency.

Individuals who have had a vegan diet for many years may develop vitamin B_{12} deficiency if they are not careful to include yeast extract in their diets. Soya milk fortified with calcium or sesame paste (Tahini) provides calcium normally obtained from cow's milk. Vitamin D is a fat-soluble vitamin. It can be manufactured by the body and half an hours' exposure of the hands and face to the sun daily is sufficient, even in winter, to enable the body to manufacture vitamin D. Older people consuming a vegan diet, who do not go out of doors, are at risk of vitamin D deficiency. All margarine has vitamin D added and eating three slices of bread spread with margarine each day will supply an individual with sufficient Vitamin D.

Meeting the dietary needs of ethnic minorities

Government statistics indicate that only 2% of older people come from minority ethnic communities. Older people from these backgrounds are less likely to enter nursing homes than older people from the host population. This may be because few services are tailored to their needs[10]. Older people from all backgrounds should be offered a diet similar to that which they would choose to eat at home. This diet should reflect religious and ethnic background.

Jewish people do not eat pork or shellfish. Some Jewish people maintain a strict Kosher diet and have separate areas within their kitchen for preparing dairy foods and meat. Separate crockery and utensils are also used for dairy foods and meat. All food is prepared by people of the Jewish faith.

Most nursing homes lack the facilities to prepare Kosher food; in many cases the individual's family wish to bring it in. Ready-prepared Kosher meals are available through the Kosher meals service in many areas of the UK. The local hospital dietician can provide details as hospitals obtain Kosher meals in this way.

Older people of the Jewish faith who do not observe a strict Kosher diet usually do not eat pork or shellfish and do not consume meat and dairy products at one sitting. In practice this may mean that the individual eats roast beef, roast potatoes and vegetables followed by apple pie, but does not have custard because it contains milk, and has a cup of tea without milk.

Older people of the Muslim faith do not eat pork. Strict Muslims eat meat which has been killed in a special way so that all blood is drained from it; This is known as Halal meat. It is possible to obtain Halal meat from Halal butchers, and it can be prepared for eating normally. If it is not possible to obtain Halal meat strict Muslims may wish to avoid meat.

Individuals who follow the Hindu faith do not eat beef. Some Hindus are vegetarian and do not eat any animal products. They follow a vegan diet as outlined earlier in this chapter.

Assessing nutritional status

Weighing an older person provides the nurse with an indication of weight. Oedema can mask the fact that an older person is underweight. It can be difficult to measure height in some older people because of age related changes and disease. If an older person is unable to stand up, a measuring tape can be used to measure them lying down in bed. Weight charts can enable the nurse to check that weight and height are in proportion. Urine should be checked for glucose and a haemoccult test carried out to eliminate the possibility of gastro-intestinal bleeding.

The individual who appears malnourished should be examined by their doctor, who may take blood to check full blood count, urea and electrolytes, and arrange serum albumen and thyroid function tests to determine the cause of malnutrition. Any underlying medical condition which is contributing to the malnutrition is treated.

A nursing history enables the nurse to identify problems which have contributed to weight loss, and to use a problem solving approach to enable the individual to enjoy a balanced diet.

The role of dietary supplements

Older people who are malnourished should be offered large helpings of normal food, and should also be offered nutritious snacks. Some older people are unable to eat enough to meet their dietary needs, and dietary supplements should be considered. The nurse should ask the individual's doctor to contact the community dietician; they cannot accept referrals from nurses. The dietician will visit the individual to assess the diet eaten and discuss dietary preferences with the individual. Dieticians usually bring samples which the individual can taste. The dietician will then recommend a range of dietary supplements which can be prescribed by the individual's doctor.

There are ranges of flavoured drinks which are high in calories and have added vitamins and mineral. Some are fruit flavoured and can be given through the day instead of water or squash. Other drinks are milk based and available in a variety of flavours. High protein puddings are also available and can be given as snacks. A number of dietary supplements are available as tasteless white powders and these can be mixed into food to provide additional calories.

Dietary supplements can be prescribed for individuals suffering from dysphagia and a range of other conditions. Details can be obtained from the latest issue of the *British National Formulary*.

High fibre diets and their role in preventing constipation

Constipation becomes more common as adults age. Disorders of the gastro-intestinal tract, such as irritable colon syndrome, haemorrhoids and anal fissure, can lead to constipation. Neurological problems, such as dementia, stroke, Parkinson's disease and disseminated sclerosis, can also lead to constipation. Endocrine disorders and prescribed medications such as iron, antacids and analgesics can contribute to constipation. Factors such as lack of exercise, immobility, inadequate fluid intake and pain can also cause it.

Nursing practice can contribute to constipation. Nurses must examine practice within their workplace and ensure that older people have sufficient time and privacy to open their bowels.

Many practitioners suggest that constipation in older people should not be treated with an increase in dietary fibre[11]. Laxatives and suppositories or enemas are recommended[12] because it is thought that a high fibre diet can cause the rectum to become loaded with soft faeces.

The dosage of laxatives, however, can be extremely difficult to calculate. Osmotic softeners which are often used to treat constipation in older people can cause the rectum to become loaded with soft faeces and individuals can leak soft faeces. Irritant laxatives can cause abdominal pain, cramp and diarrhoea, and can lead to faecal incontinence.

Introducing high fibre foods gradually into an older person's diet can eliminate the need for laxatives in many older people and contribute to general wellbeing. It is often thought that a diet is magically transformed into a high fibre diet by adding tablespoons of bran to porridge or soup. Any sensible older person will refuse food which has had bran stirred in.

High fibre foods such as bran flakes, Weetabix, Shredded Wheat and muesli can be offered as alternatives to cornflakes. Prunes, apricots and fruit compote provide additional fibre, vitamins and nutrients. Wholemeal bread high in fibre and B vitamins is a tasty alternative to sliced white bread. Cakes, crumbles and pastries can be made with 50% wholemeal flour. Many cakes such as banana cake and date loaf provide additional fibre and taste delicious. Digestive biscuits, wholemeal shortbread and wholemeal cookies with added nuts and raisins can be offered instead of custard creams. Lentils, barley and pulses can be added to soups and casseroles.

Eating a diet rich in fibre can be enjoyable and in many cases cures constipation and reduces the need for laxatives. Some older people do not wish to eat wholemeal bread or cereals high in fibre but benefit from other fibre rich foods introduced subtly into their diet[13].

It is essential that individuals who are consuming a diet rich in natural fibre drink at least two litres of fluid each day. Offering extra cups of tea, water, squash and fruit juice helps ensure that fluid intake is adequate.

Reduced fibre diets and their role in managing bowel problems

Some older people who suffer from diarrhoea benefit from a high fibre diet. The fibre absorbs excess water and the stool is more formed than before. In others this is ineffective. Some older people who are profoundly disabled, perhaps because of neurological disease, develop faecal incontinence. Helping the individual to the toilet after breakfast, when the gastro-colic reflex is at its strongest, often results in a bowel action. Such nursing interventions can prevent faecal incontinence in many extremely disabled cognitively impaired older people. Some older people, though, remain faecally incontinent. In these individuals a high fibre diet can result in the bowel becoming loaded with soft faeces, and continual leakage can occur. A low residue diet normally results in constipation which can be treated with suppositories or a mini-enema.

Further information

It is important that nurses work with the chefs or cooks employed in the home to ensure that older people's dietary needs are met. Hospital and community dieticians often run courses designed for catering staff who prepare meals for older people in local authority (part three) residential and nursing homes. These courses can be one day or may run over a series of weeks or months. The local dietician will be able to advise staff about such courses.

Nurses should work with catering staff and be willing to advise and help if staff are unsure about any aspect of an individual's diet. Some Social Services Departments (SSDs) produce books which provide dietary information, sample menus and recipes especially drawn up to meet the nutritional needs of older people living in homes. These books are normally loose-leafed plastic files and each recipe is laminated in plastic. Recipes are given which are suitable for individuals who require diabetic, high fibre, low salt, vegetarian and other diets.

The local dietician will be able to inform nurses about how to obtain such books. Relatives and friends of older people often bring fruit, biscuits and sweets as gifts when they visit. Some relatives do not understand how important it can be for an individual who suffers from diabetes, for example, to adhere to a diabetic diet. Other relatives wish to bring gifts or ask the individual home for tea or Sunday lunch and ask the nurse for information on diet. Normally the local dietician has a range of leaflets; some provide detailed dietary guidance and have been produced for nurses; others have been produced to provide information for individuals and their families. Older people who do not understand what foods should be eaten or avoided on a diet will be unable to comply with dietary advice. The nurse should obtain copies of patient information leaflets either from the local dietician or from relevant organizations such as the British Diabetic Association. Individuals requiring special diets should be given the relevant information leaflet. Relatives and friends can also be given copies and this will help them to ensure that food provided as gifts or at home when the older person visits is appropriate to the diet.

Conclusion

The nurse can help ensure that older people are provided with a diet which meets their needs and consists of the type of foods which would be chosen at home. Providing suitable cutlery and aids can enable older people to retain independence. Providing snacks reduces the risk that some older people will suffer from underfeeding.

Identifying any difficulties an older person has in eating enables the nurse to adopt a problem solving approach and to provide care tailored to the individual's needs. The nurse has a duty to ensure that the older person's dietary needs are met. The nurse can ask the individual's doctor to investigate any medical causes of malnutrition and prescribe treatment wherever possible, referring to dieticians if required. The nurse can work with other professionals, such as clinical nurse specialists and speech and language therapists, to ensure that an individual's needs are met.

Useful addresses and telephone numbers

Local dietician

Local diabetic nurse specialist

Further information

The British Diabetic Association produce a catalogue and can provide information and advice on diabetes:

The British Diabetic Association
10 Queen Anne Street
London W1M 0BD
Tel. 0171 323 1531

The Vegetarian Society provides a useful leaflet, *Healthy Nutrition in Later Life*, available free if SAE enclosed. They also offer nutritional advice:

The Vegetarian Society
Park Dale
Dunham Road
Altringham
Cheshire
WA14 4QG
Tel 0161 928 0793

References

(1) Department of Health and Social Security (1979) *Nutrition and Health in Old Age*. Reports on health and social subjects no 16. HMSO, London.

(2) Department of Health (1991) *Dietary Reference Values for food, energy and nutrients for the United Kingdom*. Report on health and social subjects no 41. HMSO, London.

(3) Department of Health (1991) Committee on Medical Aspects of Food Policy. Working group on nutrition of elderly people. HMSO, London.

(4) Prentice, A.M. (1988) Is severe wasting in elderly mental patients caused by excessive energy requirement? *Age & Ageing*, 18, 158–67.

(5) Heath, M.R. (1972) Dietary selection by elderly persons related to dental state. *British Dental Journal*, 132, 145–8.

(6) *General Household Survey* (1992) Table no 3.1 and figures 3A-3C. HMSO, London.

(7) Hatton, P. (1990) Primum non nocere – an analysis of drugs prescribed to elderly patients in private nursing homes registered with Harrogate Health Authority. *Care of the Elderly*, **2** (4) 166–8.

(8) Nazarko, L. (1993) Nutritional problems in nursing homes. *Nursing Standard*, **7** (27) 33–6.

(9) Brastow, M.D. *et al.* (1983) Benefits of supplementary feeding after fractured neck of femur; a randomised control trial. *British Medical Journal*, 287, 1589–92.

(10) Norman, A. (1988) Triple Jeopardy: *Growing Old in a Second Homeland*. Centre for Policy on Ageing, London.

(11) Ardron, M.E. & Main, A.N.H. (1990) Management of constipation. *British Medical Journal*, 300, 1400.

(12) Roe, B. & Williams, K. (1994) *Clinical Handbook for Continence Care*. Scutari Press, Harrow.

(13) Nazarko, L. (1993) Preventing Constipation. *Elderly Care*, **5** (2) 32–3.

Chapter 11
Obtaining Services

Introduction

Department of Health guidance states clearly that older people living in nursing homes have the same right to health services as people living in their own homes. Some individuals managing services appear not to be aware of this guidance. Nurses, in some areas, experience great difficulty in obtaining access to services on behalf of older people who require them. It is the responsibility of the nurse to be aware of services available. The aim of this chapter is to outline services available and give nurses information which will enable them to organize these services when required.

Chiropody services

Age related changes may make older people's nails difficult to cut. Many older people have very tough thickened toe nails. This is because reduced blood supply to the nails causes changes in the nail bed. Regular cutting of toe nails is important and prevents problems such as ingrowing toe nails. Many older people experience difficulty in cutting their own toe nails because they are unable to bend down or lack the co-ordination to cut nails. Many nurses have never cut toe nails during their nursing careers and a myth has grown up that nurses do not carry out this task. There is no reason why nurses should not cut older people's toe nails.

It is often impossible to cut them with ordinary nail scissors normally used to cut finger nails. Each nursing home should purchase suitable equipment to enable nurses to cut toe nails. A strong pair of toe nail clippers, a pair of toe nail scissors and a selection of files and emery boards are required. It is usually easier to cut tough thickened toe nails after the individual has had a soak in a warm bath, as this softens the nails. Nails should be cut straight across and any rough edges filed with a nail file or emery board.

Nurses can also cut toe nails in older people who suffer from diabetes.

Older people who are suffering from vascular problems should be referred to a chiropodist for treatment.

Some older people suffer from corns, bunions, ingrowing toe nails and other problems outside the nurse's sphere of competence. Individuals suffering from such problems should be referred to a chiropodist for treatment.

Obtaining chiropody services

Community based chiropodists are often based at the local hospital. They work with foot-care assistants to provide services. Chiropodists normally visit housebound older people at home to carry out treatment. Mobile older people are often asked to visit community chiropody clinics, which chiropodists hold in local health centres.

The numbers of older people requiring community chiropody services have increased enormously in recent years. Greater numbers of older people are now living in nursing and residential homes. In many areas, though, chiropody services have not expanded to take account of the greater numbers of people requiring chiropody. Many chiropodists now find that they are able to see older people less frequently than before. An older person who was receiving chiropody services every six weeks may now only receive services every eight weeks.

Nurses can contact their local chiropody department and request chiropody treatment for the older people in the home. The chiropody department will probably send a foot-care assistant for a few hours every eight weeks. It will not be possible for each older person to have nails cut during this session. Staff shortages or illness can mean that a session is missed. If nurses carry out routine footcare and nail cutting for the majority of older people living in the nursing home, the chiropodist or foot-care assistant can concentrate on the individuals who require specialist treatment.

If the nurse does not feel confident about cutting older people's toe nails or would like advice about purchasing suitable nail clippers and cutters, advice and help can be obtained from the local chiropodist. Many chiropodists welcome nurses to their foot-care clinics and will spend a few hours helping the nurse become proficient at cutting what initially appear to be uncuttable thickened toe nails.

Contact number of local chiropodist

Emergency chiropody

Foot problems seldom occur on the day of the chiropodist's visit. Older people can develop ingrowing toe nails which can be painful and require prompt treatment. Bunions can become painful and infected. An individual can have an accident which leads to bleeding under the nail. Nails can become caught, torn and damaged. In such cases the nurse should contact the chiropodist, who may be able to visit the home that day to offer emergency treatment. Nurses who carry out routine foot-care and have developed a good relationship with the chiropodist normally find chiropodists are willing to visit immediately.

Sometimes the chiropodist may suggest that the older person is brought to a nearby health centre if a clinic is in progress. The nurse who recognizes the chiropodist as a fellow professional and builds a good working relationship will find that access to chiropody services is not difficult.

Private chiropody

NHS chiropodists often lack the time to visit frequently enough to ensure that all older people living within the nursing home have their nails cut on a regular basis. Nurses are often approached by private chiropodists offering nail cutting sessions. In some homes this charge is paid by older people themselves; in others the home bears the cost. The charges for private chiropody vary but rates from £8 to £15 per patient are not uncommon. It normally takes 10 to 15 minutes to cut an older person's nails and file any rough edges.

Specialist footwear and appliances

Many older people suffer from disabilities and specialist footwear and appliances can make a real difference to an individual's quality of life. Many older people enter nursing homes after sustaining falls which have resulted in fracture. Surgical treatment of fractured femurs usually involves pinning and plating of the femur. In some cases total hip replacements are carried out. Such surgery often results in the ligaments on the affected leg becoming stretched. The result is that the individual has one leg longer than the other. Older people who fail to make a rapid recovery are often discharged to nursing homes immobile.

The nurse can ask the individual's doctor to complete a referral form and send this to the surgical appliance department, which is usually based at the local hospital. The older person will either be visited at the home or given an appointment to see the orthotist. The orthotist measures both legs and orders specially-made shoes which accom-modate any shortening. Providing shoes to correct shortening can make a real difference to an older person's life. It becomes possible for the individual to regain mobility and independence.

Older people who have suffered strokes often suffer from feet and ankles which tend to turn inwards or outwards (talipes equinus or talipes varus). These foot deformities hamper walking and increase the risk of falls. The orthotist is often able to correct such problems by providing shoes with a wedge on one part of the sole. In other cases the orthotist may arrange for a calliper to be provided. The older person's own shoes are sometimes adapted to accommodate a calliper; in other cases shoes and a calliper are supplied.

Some older people suffer from foot deformities such as large bunions and hammer toes. It can be impossible to find shoes to fit and so the older person wears large, wide ill-fitting carpet slippers. These can so easily contribute to accidents and falls. Some older people suffer from oedema, which prevents them wearing shoes. They tend to wear slippers and in some cases cut the slippers at the front to give them more room. These slippers can easily fall off during walking. The orthotist can provide special shoes to accommodate foot deformities and oedema. These shoes fit properly, make walking more comfortable and reduce the risk of accidents.

Some older people suffer from osteo-arthritis and when this affects the knee joints they can be painful and can tend to 'give'. This can result in falls. The orthotist can supply knee supports which support arthritic knees and reduce pain on walking.

Older people who have suffered from strokes should be encouraged to exercise hemiplegic or weakened limbs. The nurse should carry out a range of passive movements to affected limbs when an older person is unable to do this. Relatives can also be encouraged to assist in carrying out passive movements. Some older people's limbs tend to contract despite exercise and passive movement and can easily become deformed. Hands can become tightly clenched and wrists turned inwards. Such deformities can cause older people intense pain.

The individual's doctor may prescribe muscle relaxants in such cases but these are not always effective and can cause unpleasant side effects such as urinary incontinence (by relaxing the detrusor muscle which controls the bladder) or drowsiness. The orthotist can examine the individual and provide an appropriate splint for the hand or the hand and wrist. There are a number of different types; some, known as 'lively splints', enable the individual to use the hand whilst wearing the splint.

Splints can be worn only at night or when the patient is not exercising. The orthotist will advise nurses about the use of each splint on each patient. Splints can reduce pain, prevent deformity, reduce or eliminate the need for drugs which can have troublesome side effects, and make a real difference to an older person's quality of life.

Oedema can easily occur in older people who are unable to walk or who are not encouraged and helped to walk. Postural oedema is often treated with diuretics but these can predispose an older person to urinary incontinence; the fear of urinary incontinence can lead older people to become depressed and can reduce mobility. This can lead to a vicious cycle where more drugs are prescribed to treat symptoms.

Older people who suffer from postural oedema should be encouraged and assisted to walk whenever possible. If oedema persists despite mobilisation, where possible, and elevation, the orthotist can measure the individual for surgical stockings. Support stockings are available in four levels of compression from light to extra high. They should be used to prevent recurrence of leg ulcers in individuals who have suffered from varicose ulcers; details are given in Chapter 6. Support stockings are available in a range of colours and the individual can choose the colour she prefers. It is important to ensure that the patient chooses a colour she is happy to wear, otherwise she may not wear them when they arrive. Men are reluctant to wear stockings! Knee length support stockings are available in black and are indistinguishable from men's knee length socks. The nurse who refers to them as support socks may find male patients wear them more readily.

Many orthotists now only supply one pair of support stockings. The measurements are left with the nurse (and kept on record at surgical appliances) so that further supplies can be ordered from the local pharmacist on FP10 prescription.

Hairdressing

Most older women enjoyed going to the hairdresser for a weekly or fortnightly hairdo before admission to the home. Having a shampoo and set or a perm is a real morale booster for most older women. Nursing homes normally have a hairdresser who visits regularly, usually weekly. The hairdresser provides a full range of services. In many homes patients pay the hairdresser for this service; prices are usually lower than in local salons.

Some patients may prefer to visit a local salon and may require the nurse's help to arrange an appointment and get to and from the salon.

Wigs

Losing hair is one of the most traumatic experiences an older woman can suffer. Some older women have undergone chemotherapy whilst others may have suffered from hair loss as a result of undetected thyroid disease. NHS wigs can be supplied and worn until the hair regrows. A wig can make a tremendous difference to morale and the nurse should never assume that just because a woman is in her 80s or 90s she no longer cares how she looks.

Obtaining specialist services

All the appliances described can be obtained from the surgical appliances department of the local hospital. Normally the individual's doctor writes a referral note which is sent to the department. A letter from a consultant may be required stating the reason for hair loss if a wig is required. GPs are very busy and they can often find it difficult to find the time to write referral letters for appliances. It may be helpful if the home prepares a standard letter. The doctor can then fill in the blank spaces with details of the patient and the type of appliance required, and sign the letter. Hospitals deal with huge volumes of mail and from time to time letters fail to reach their destination. Keeping a photocopy of referrals in the patient's notes ensures that if this happens another copy of the referral can be sent to the hospital. This saves the nurse's time as she does not have to obtain another letter, and she ensures that the patient is seen as quickly as possible.

Many hospitals employ orthotists on a sessional basis and prefer to see people at their outpatient clinics. Individuals attending outpatient clinics will require hospital transport (unless the home has its own transport facilities); using hospital transport can involve long delays waiting for it. This can be exhausting, especially for individuals who have recently undergone major surgery or suffered strokes. It is good practice for the home to send a member of staff to accompany an individual attending an outpatient appointment.

Domiciliary visits can be arranged and if a number of individuals require appliances, domiciliary visits are more cost effective than the hospital budget bearing the costs of both transport and the orthotist's time.

Surgical appliances are provided free of charge to older people. The costs of the appliances, the orthotist's salary and hospital transport required to take individuals to clinics, all come from the hospital budget. In the future fundholding GPs will be required to purchase these services from hospitals. Appliances such as shoes and splints may appear expensive to budget conscious GP fundholders, and the nurse may have to remind doctors that such services reduce the need for expensive drugs, and improve an older person's wellbeing.

Ophthalmic services

Few older people have perfect vision; government statistics indicate that 96% of people over the age of 75 wear glasses[1]. The nurse who has perfect vision may not appreciate the importance of an older person having regular eye tests and obtaining spectacles which provide the best possible correction. An older person who has lost their glasses or who has glasses which are no longer appropriate can be at risk of falling. Eating may become difficult. Choosing clothes from the wardrobe may become difficult; dressing can become a struggle. It may no longer be possible to enjoy reading books or daily newspapers. Moving freely around the home can become difficult. The older person who can no longer read the time, read signs, read papers or watch television can easily become disorientated and distressed.

Some older people who enter the home may have been attending one particular optician for many years. If the optician is local, the older person should continue to receive eye care from them. This ensures continuity of care. In some cases the older person does not have a local optician or has not visited an optician in many years. The home should arrange for an optician to provide optical services for older people living in the home.

There are two different types of opticians:

(1) ophthalmic opticians are qualified to examine eyes and detect the presence of disease and also to test sight, prescribe and dispense spectacles to correct visual problems
(2) dispensing opticians are qualified to dispense and fit spectacles but not to examine eyes for abnormalities or to test vision and prescribe spectacles.

The home should make arrangements with an ophthalmic optician to provide services to the home. Ophthalmic opticians are independent practitioners. They receive fees from the NHS for providing optical services to individuals who are eligible for NHS ophthalmic services. Individuals who are not eligible for these are charged for ophthalmic services.

There are usually a number of opticians within an area and the nurse can choose which one to arrange services with. Ideally the optician should be located near the home, if possible within walking distance. This makes trips to the opticians more convenient. The optician should have a flexible appointments system and it should be possible to arrange an appointment quickly. If an optician cannot offer an appointment within 48 hours, then choose another optician. It is important to check how quickly an optician can obtain glasses in an emergency. If an older person who is dependent on glasses damages them, it is important to obtain new glasses quickly. Some opticians can obtain new glasses within 24 hours or less, others can take three weeks.

An optician who values the custom of older people resident at the nursing home will normally carry out minor repairs without charge. Some opticians feel that their work is completed when glasses are dispensed. It is important that the individual tries on glasses to ensure they fit correctly; the optician can make any adjustments to ensure the best possible fit at this stage.

If an older person is too frail or unwell to leave the home the optician can make a domiciliary visit. It is preferable to examine eyes at the optician's fully-equipped surgery, and domiciliary visits should only be requested if absolutely necessary. Some opticians choose to visit the home and fit spectacles when they are ready, as it is more convenient for an older person to have the fitting at the home. Opticians do not charge for fitting visits.

Eye tests should be carried out each year. The optician will normally have a system which sends out annual reminders to patients advising them that their next eye test is due. An eye test normally takes half an hour. Individuals should be escorted to the opticians and a list of medications and details of medical history should be given, as the optician will wish to take a medical history. The member of staff who escorts the older person may have to help the individual get into the examining chair.

The optician examines the older person's eyes, and may detect signs of eye abnormality or disease. If any abnormality or disease is detected the optician will write details of his findings on a green form. This form will be given to the older person or the escort. The nurse should photocopy the form and retain the copy in the individual's notes. The original should be given to the individual's GP who will refer to the ophthalmology department of the local hospital. If the optician detects eye disease which requires urgent treatment, such as acute glaucoma, detached retina or retinal haemorrhage, they will normally contact the hospital direct and have the patient sent there immediately.

Some opticians offer specialist 'low vision' services which aim to help maximize the vision of people with severe sight defects. Opticians can advise and arrange to supply magnifying glasses, including some with lights, and other aids to vision.

Mobile opticians

Some opticians are now specializing in caring for older people living in nursing and residential homes and are offering a mobile optician's service. The optician has a large, fully-equipped vehicle which is driven to the nursing home. All individuals requiring eye tests are seen and examined in the vehicle, which carries a full range of frames; individuals can choose frames and order spectacles. The vehicle returns when spectacles are ready and all individuals have their spectacles fitted. Opticians offering such services usually offer free eye tests to individuals who are not eligible for NHS eye tests.

Nurses working in rural areas find mobile optician's services very useful. Every visit is a domiciliary visit and such services save time. Many city and suburban areas are now served by mobile opticians. They normally make regular visits to the nursing home, usually every three months. Older people who have broken their glasses, who have been admitted to the home between visits or are experiencing problems seeing, should not have to wait weeks or months until the next visit to obtain services. It is important for the nurse to check what arrangements mobile opticians make to provide ad hoc services, before making arrangements with them to provide ophthalmic services to the home.

NHS and private eye tests and spectacles

Older people who are receiving income support are eligible for free NHS eye tests. Older people who have savings in excess of £8000 are charged for eye tests. Individuals who suffer from diabetes or who have a close family member who has suffered from glaucoma are eligible for free NHS eye tests regardless of income. Private eye tests normally cost £12 to £15. Domiciliary eye tests are available free to those eligible for NHS eye tests, but individuals who are not eligible are normally charged a fee of £25 in addition to the cost of the eye test. Some opticians offer free eye tests to individuals who buy spectacles from them. The nurse may be able to negotiate such a scheme with the optician, on behalf of the patients.

Individuals on income support are given financial help with the costs of glasses, on a voucher scheme. A voucher is available towards the cost of frames and is worth either £25 or £39.30, depending on the frames required. A voucher is also available towards the cost of lenses. This is normally £44. It is usually possible for an older person on income support to obtain an attractive pair of glasses using the vouchers without having to pay any money towards the cost. Individuals may choose to have more expensive frames if they wish, and meet the additional costs.

Individuals who are not on income support do not receive any financial help towards the cost of glasses.

It is possible to have the individual's name engraved inside the arm of glasses. This can help identify glasses when they are put down and forgotten. Many opticians will provide this service free of charge if requested.

Some older people require glasses for close and distance work. In some cases bifocal glasses are prescribed, but these can be difficult to use: in order to see close up the individual must look out of the bottom half of the glasses and in order to see in the distance the individual must look out of the top half of the glasses. If an individual looks out of the wrong part the vision is poor.

Some people (young and old) are unable to cope with bifocal glasses and may require reading and distance glasses. Older people who require two sets of glasses should be advised to choose different frames or different coloured frames to avoid confusion. The optician can engrave an R for reading or D for distance on the inner arm of the glasses, in case the older person or staff mix up the two pairs.

Further information

The British College of Optometrists produces two useful leaflets: *Choosing an Optician* and *Domiciliary Eye Care Services – Guidance for managers of residential care and nursing homes*. The College can provide information and advise on ophthalmic services.

> The British College of Optometrists
> 10 Knaresborough Place
> London SW5 OTG.
> Tel. 0171 373 7765.

The Department of Health provides information on eligibility for NHS eye tests and details of voucher systems, in patient information leaflet G11. This is available from opticians and GP's surgeries.

Useful name and address

Local optician

Dental services

Most older people wear dentures or partial dentures, while some older people retain their natural teeth. It is important that the home has made arrangements to provide patients with dental care. Some older people are registered with local dentists and should be encouraged to continue to obtain treatment from their dentist. This ensures continuity of care. Some older people may have moved to the area to be near family and friends. The home should make arrangements to ensure that dental services are available for older people who require them.

Dental services can either be obtained from a dental surgeon who is in practice locally or from the NHS community dentist. Many independent dental surgeons are willing to provide dental services to older people but are no longer taking on new NHS patients. In some parts of the UK it can be extremely difficult to find a dentist willing to offer NHS treatment. A list of dentists is available from the local library and the nurse can phone and ask if dentists are prepared to offer NHS dental services.

Although some dentists are willing to offer these services they may not be willing to make new dentures for NHS patients. Nurses should clarify this point before considering referring patients to the dentist, as dentures supplied privately cost from £250 to £300. Many older people living in nursing homes, who are on income support, are unable to afford to pay for private dentures.

If the nurse is unable to find a dentist offering NHS services to new patients she can contact the local Family Services Health Authority (FSHA) who will be able to find a dentist. The dentist(s) offering such services may be some distance away, and this is an important consideration as transport may be required to take individuals to appointments, and escorts may be absent from the home for a considerable time. It can be difficult to organize prompt emergency treatment in such circumstances. Some older people may require domiciliary treatment and dentists may be unwilling to travel considerable distances to offer it.

NHS community dentists are employed directly by NHS community trusts to provide dental services to individuals living in the community. They provide services in local health centres and offer domiciliary services. Community dentists usually provide specialized dental care to children with special needs and people with learning disability living in the community, as well as other client groups. They normally have a greater expertise in dealing with disabled and cognitively impaired individuals, and can offer a greater range of dental techniques developed to help such individuals.

Community dentists will visit older people in nursing homes and provide all dental care for individuals living in the home. Community dentists normally work with a trained dental nurse and a hygienist. Most dental treatments are carried out within the home. The community dentist carries out routine dental examinations and works with the hygienist and dental nurse to provide older people and nurses with advice and help to ensure good oral hygiene and dental care.

Community dentists, unfortunately, are extremely busy and whilst they provide a superb emergency service, they may have to place older people on a waiting list for dentures. It may be six or eight weeks before the dentist can begin taking impressions and order dentures.

Older people are not charged for any treatment or dentures supplied by community dentists; the costs are borne by the community trust. Individuals who require new dentures and are unwilling to wait, but can afford to pay, may prefer to pay a local dentist for private treatment.

The local hospital or community NHS trust will be able to supply the telephone number of the community dentist for your area.

Useful address and telephone number

Dentist

Hearing aids services

Causes of hearing problems

Hearing loss affects 17% of the adult population and at least 50% of older people living in nursing homes. The commonest cause of hearing loss is wax in the ears. Wax is often visible in the outer ear. Simple treatment such as ear drops or warm olive oil can be put in the ears three times a day for three to five days. This softens the wax and the ears can then be syringed. The patient's doctor should be asked to check that the ears are completely free of wax.

If hearing loss persists the older person's doctor should be asked to refer to the ENT clinic at the local hospital so that hearing can be checked by carrying out an audiogram. NHS waiting lists for audiograms can be lengthy and some older people have to wait six months for an initial appointment. It is important to ensure that ears are clear of wax prior to an audiogram. If the older person's ears are blocked with wax it is impossible to carry out an audiogram and the nurse is asked to make a further appointment after the wax has been removed.

Hearing aids

Older people who suffer from hearing loss are often supplied with hearing aids. The nurse may assume that hearing aids enable individuals to hear normally. Hearing aids in fact amplify sounds and make them louder.

The nurse should ensure that staff and relatives are aware of the actions they can take to help older people with hearing difficulties to hear. It is important not to shout, as this distorts the voice. People should face the individual and speak slowly and clearly. Plain language should be used and gestures can be used if an individual has difficulty hearing. It is important to cut out background noise, closing doors, turning down the television or closing the window to shut out traffic noise, can help people with hearing impairment to hear.

Older people who do not wear their hearing aids

Some older people do not wear their hearing aids. If they lost their hearing gradually, a hearing aid suddenly exposes them to a great deal of noise, which they may find unbearable. But if they do not use the hearing aid they become cut off from normal life and unable to communicate. The nurse should encourage older people to wear their hearing aids. Suggest that the older person wears the aid twice a day for an hour and gradually encourage it to be used at all times. This allows them to get used to our noisy world again.

Some older people find it difficult to put the mould in their ear and to work the controls, but may not wish to ask for help. Nurses should be sensitive to such problems and offer help in a tactful way.

Hearing aids – common problems

Many hearing aids fail to work because the batteries are dead. There are two types of hearing aid batteries available for NHS aids which fit behind the ear. The normal battery will normally last for three or four days if the hearing aid is turned off when the older person goes to sleep. If the aid is left on, the battery will only last for a day or two. Long life batteries normally last about a week if used during waking hours.

Hearing aid batteries are supplied in small blister packs. A dozen ordinary batteries or eight long-life batteries are usually supplied. Unused batteries have a small blue sticker on them which must be removed before use. Occasionally older people and staff open the blister pack and remove the blue stickers; used and unused batteries can then become mixed up. The only way to check batteries when the stickers have been removed is to ask the individual to remove the aid. Place a battery in the aid and turn it up to the highest setting; charged batteries will cause the aid to oscillate and emit a high pitched screeching sound. Charged batteries can then be remarked with sticky tape or labels.

Changing hearing aid batteries is a fiddly task and many older people find this difficult; the nurse should offer help if required.

Hearing aids whistle and oscillate at times. Oscillating aids are not functioning properly and the nurse should check them. The commonest cause of oscillation is that the aid is turned up too high, turning it down so that the whistling ceases but the individual is able to hear, is often all that is required. If the aid continues to oscillate even on a low setting such as one or two, the nurse should ask the individual to remove the aid and should check the plastic tube which connects to the ear mould. The tube should be slightly opaque, white and flexible; if it has hardened or yellowed it should be replaced. Spare tubing is supplied with all aids and the nurse cuts a length to size and replaces it. Tubing should normally be changed every two months.

The nurse should also check the mould which fits in the patient's ear. Wax often builds up in the ear drum behind the mould and a small piece of wax can block the mould and cause oscillation. Wax can be removed from the mould with a needle or safely pin. The mould can then be washed in warm water, reconnected to the aid and returned.

If wax has blocked the mould, the ears should be checked for wax; any build up should be removed using ear drops and syringing. If the aid continues to oscillate it is possible that the ear mould no longer fits properly and a new mould is required. The nurse can contact the audiology clinic direct and make an appointment for the individual to be seen.

Individuals who are issued with hearing aids are supplied with a small brown hearing aid book. This book contains details of the type of aid, batteries and tube supplied, and gives the address of the local audiology clinic. When further supplies of batteries are required (usually when half of the supplied batteries have been used) the used batteries are returned to the audiology department with the book and a request for further batteries and tubing; this can be done by post. It is important to return used batteries as these are recharged.

Useful address and telephone number

Hearing aid department

Further information

Counsel and Care produce a free fact sheet (number 21), *Helping Residents to Hear*. This can be obtained by sending an SAE. They have also produced a study on the needs of older people with hearing loss living in residential and nursing homes. This provides guidance on caring for individuals who have hearing difficulties. It is called *Sound Barriers* and costs £5 from the address below.

Counsel and Care
Twyman House
16, Bonny Street
London NW1 9PG.
Telephone: 0171 485 1566 (10.30 AM to 4 PM).

Conclusion

Older people may require aids of some kind to prevent deformity developing after illness. Many older people require aids to enable them to walk, see, hear and eat. Older people are often unaware of the range of aids and services available to enable them to participate fully in life. The nurse can work with older people to identify needs, and can then work with other professionals to ensure that these needs are met and older people are able to enjoy a greater degree of independence.

Reference

(1) *General Household Survey* (1992) Table no 3, 25. HMSO, London.

Chapter 12
Rehabilitation

Introduction

Older people often enter nursing homes at their lowest ebb, following a major life crisis. Illness, accident or the loss of a loved one can cause them to enter nursing home care. They have usually been moved from home to hospital to nursing home. Although efforts have been made to help heal physical damage they have often had little help in coming to terms mentally with a major life event. Older people who enter nursing homes have 'failed' to get better. Many have low expectations of themselves and of the nursing home; most older people would, given a choice, prefer to live at home, and some individuals feel that others have given up on them and transferred them to the nursing home to await death. Life can seem hopeless and worthless to some older people when they enter a nursing home[1].

Many older people admitted to nursing homes have the potential to be rehabilitated and can, with skilled care from a nurse-led multi-disciplinary team either return home or enjoy an enhanced quality of life within the nursing home.

In the past, older people spent longer in hospital[2]. Now the average stay following a cerebrovascular accident has fallen to three weeks. An older person who has suffered a fractured femur is now normally treated surgically and the femur is pinned and plated. The average stay following this is now ten days. These extremely short hospital stays seldom give older people an opportunity to complete the process of healing mind and body after a major illness. The majority of older people admitted to nursing homes are admitted from hospital.

Older people admitted from hospital are much more dependent than they were before. Most are immobile or have extremely limited mobility[3] and many suffer from uninvestigated and untreated urinary incontinence. Many have pressure sores. Entering a nursing home is a traumatic experience for them. Many feel depressed and unhappy, especially at the thought of having to give up their home and enter a nursing home.

The goal of skilled nursing care is to prevent or reverse 'excess

151

disability' and ensure that the patient is not prematurely disabled and is enabled to function to capacity. The aims of rehabilitation are to enable the older person to recover from the major life event which necessitated their admission to the nursing home. In many cases a full recovery and subsequent discharge is not possible. It is possible, though, to help the older person to make as full a recovery as possible. The individual who regains skills and is able to carry out some aspects of care regains a measure of independence and an enhanced quality of life.

Assessing for rehabilitation

A full assessment should be carried out prior to the older person being admitted to the nursing home; details are given in Chapter 2. On admission this assessment should be reviewed as some time may have elapsed from assessment to admission, or the patient's condition may have changed rapidly. It is helpful if a dependency score is used; details of the ENAZ dependency score are given in Chapter 2. The dependency score provides a base line assessment and it is then possible to determine progress by scoring again at a later date.

It is impossible to plan a rehabilitation programme without the consent and active participation of the patient. An extremely ill older person who has been admitted with a pressure sore may lack the will to begin a rehabilitation programme. It is important to talk to the individual and discover the individual's priorities. Basic needs such as freedom from pain, having sufficient food and fluids and being able to feel safe to express such needs are normally the older person's first priorities. It is only possible to begin working towards rehabilitation when these basic needs have been met.

The nurse, though, must plan ahead. If for example an older person has been admitted to the home immobile and suffering from a sacral pressure sore, the nurse must determine short and long term goals.

The short term goals would be to ensure that:

- pain was controlled
- psychological needs were met
- a diet with sufficient calories, protein and nutrients was offered and consumed
- pressure relieving devices were used
- an appropriate dressing was used to promote wound healing.

The long term goals may include:

- ensuring that suitable shoes are provided to correct shortening following surgery
- organizing physiotherapy to build muscle strength
- ordering a walking frame.

The nurse must work with the patient to ensure that whilst the most pressing needs are met quickly, work continues to meet long term goals. In some cases nurse and patient will have differing priorities and goals. An older person with restricted mobility who enjoys reading and has lost her glasses may view her first priority as obtaining new glasses so that she can continue to keep in touch with the world by reading the paper. The nurse's priority may be to take a wound swab and ensure that her pressure sore is not infected. The sensitive and aware nurse will balance nursing and patient priorities to ensure that individual's needs are met, and will work in partnership with the patient towards common goals. The nurse who delays organizing an optician's appointment for an older person may find that the older person becomes depressed and unwilling to eat or work with the nurse towards rehabilitation.

Barriers to rehabilitation

Nursing practice plays an important part in enabling older people to fulfil their full potential, and in preventing premature disablement and unnecessary dependence on nursing staff. Nursing can actively foster disability by discouraging older people from walking, by thoughtlessly placing obstacles in an older person's path, or by leaving walking frames, shoes and aids out of the older person's reach.

Nursing staff may encourage older people to rely on nursing staff pushing them around in wheelchairs 'because it's quicker' or because 'it must be such a struggle for poor Mary'. Some nursing staff lift older people who are able to transfer independently and insist on dressing older people who are able to dress themselves slowly. These actions undermine an older person's abilities and foster a sense of power-lessness and apathy: 'What's the sense of trying; they'll only say I did it wrong'.

It the nurse is working with an older person to enable them to regain skills, it is vital that all nursing staff are aware of the rehabilitation programme and work together to support the older person. Staff must recognize that older people, like all others, have the right to struggle to regain skills if they so wish. The older person should be offered support and help in ways that do not undermine their efforts to regain skills. The older person should not be made to feel slow or clumsy, and effort and achievement should be praised.

The manager's attitude is important to rehabilitation. A manager who stresses that beds must be made by a certain time, or baths completed by a certain time, places staff under pressure to speed up and have work completed to a fixed timescale. Staff normally respond by encouraging older people to 'hurry up', and it is so much quicker to do something for an older person rather than enable them to do it for themselves. Managers who wish to encourage older people to regain or retain self care skills must be careful to ensure that staff do not feel pressurized to have tasks completed within a set timescale.

The older person's relatives can actively undermine attempts at rehabilitation. Many relatives feel extremely guilty about their loved one living in a nursing home. Some family members can pressurize one member of the family (often a daughter or daughter-in-law) to take the older person home and provide care. Relatives in this position can feel extremely threatened by an older person regaining skills, as they may feel that staff are planning to discharge the older person to their care.

Some relatives feel that their loved one has entered a nursing home to be looked after. Nurses who encourage the older person to maintain or regain skills are, in the eyes of such relatives, failing to provide care. It is important to obtain the older person's consent and discuss the aims of any rehabilitation plan with relatives. Relatives who are aware of the advantages of rehabilitation and do not feel threatened by the older person's progress can work together with the older person, nurses and other professionals to enhance care and improve skills.

Enlisting the help of other professionals

Nurses do not possess all the skills required to help an older person rehabilitate. Nurses, though, because of the amount of patient contact they have, are in a unique position to assess the needs of an older person and to organize referral to other professionals. The older person benefits from a home where nurses co-ordinate and work with other professionals towards common goals which have been determined by the older person and the nurse.

Physiotherapy

Many older people benefit from physiotherapy, yet the pace of admission and discharge in hospitals today is so great that many have had little physiotherapy treatment during their hospital stay. The physiotherapist can advise older people on exercises which will improve muscle strength and help them regain function, or will prevent deformity following illness.

There are three methods of arranging physiotherapy services for individuals living in nursing homes. The first is to employ a part-time physiotherapist. Some homes employ one by placing an advertisement in the local paper. The salary offered for twenty hours per week is normally around £8000 to 10 000 per year. It is also possible to obtain details of physiotherapists in private practice from the local Yellow Pages. These physiotherapists typically charge from £20 to £30 for a 45 minute treatment session.

The majority of older people who live in nursing homes have their fees met either under the old DSS scheme or by local authorities under the Community Care Act. Homes where most individuals are state funded may be unable to afford to pay either a directly employed or a sessional physiotherapist. Some older people who have sufficient funds to meet their own fees may be able to afford private physiotherapy. Community physiotherapy is available from the NHS.

Nurses are unable to request physiotherapy but can ask the individual's doctor to request it. Many community trusts have a standard physiotherapy referral form which the doctor must complete. The nurse can obtain a supply of these from the local community physiotherapist and they can be kept at the home so that they are available to the individual's doctor when a referral is required. Taking a photocopy of the form and filing it in the older person's notes ensures that the nurse can readily supply a copy of the referral if the original gets lost in the post or at the community physiotherapy offices. The nurse should make sure the referral is obtained and posted off as quickly as possible. There is normally a waiting list which varies nationally from three weeks to three months for an initial assessment.

The physiotherapist normally visits and makes an initial assessment and then decides how often the individual can have treatment. Unfortunately whilst the numbers of older people living in nursing homes have increased greatly in recent years and the demands on the time of community physiotherapists have increased, there has not been a corresponding rise in the numbers of NHS community physiotherapists.

The nurse must ensure that the older person, all nursing staff and relatives if they wish to be involved, encourage and assist the older person with the physiotherapy programme. This involvement is crucial if any benefit is to be obtained from the extremely limited amount of NHS physiotherapy currently available to nursing home patients.

The limitations of nursing home based physiotherapy

Most nursing homes are small units; the average size is currently 39 beds. Average size nursing homes normally do not have the facilities which some older people require if they are to make an optimal recovery. The larger corporate nursing homes still account for only 3% of all nursing home beds, but some of them do have fully equipped physiotherapy facilities and equipment such as parallel bars.

Some older people find that their potential to regain skills is limited because equipment and resources are not available within the nursing home. It is possible in such circumstances to ask the community physiotherapist or the individual's doctor to refer to the hospital physiotherapy department. Some hospital physiotherapy departments are unenthusiastic about treating older people from nursing homes and the nurse needs to act as the older person's advocate, adopting a firm but polite stance. Nurses who are unable to obtain access for older people in such circumstances should inform the local Community Health Council (CHC) of any problems. This is seldom necessary as mere mention of the CHC normally facilitates access.

Useful addresses and telephone numbers

Local community physiotherapist

Private physiotherapist (if used)

Hospital physiotherapy department

Communication problems

Many older people who are admitted to nursing homes have communication problems. These are a common feature of neurological disease, and are commonly seen after strokes if the speech centre in the brain has been affected by the stroke. They can cause different types of problems.

Older people suffering from receptive dysphasia are unable to understand speech or make sense of the content of speech. Individuals suffering from expressive dysphasia understand every word and gesture but cannot find the right words to communicate. These individuals mix up words and may say yes instead of no or plate instead of cup. They have difficulty in expressing their needs.

Dysarthria – difficulty with articulating words – is often associated with poor muscle control. Strokes can affect the muscles of the throat, tongue, lips and face. Some older people have difficulty in swallowing after a stroke. Many older people wear dentures and these are kept in place partly by the muscles in the mouth. If these muscles are affected, dentures can slip around or can be almost impossible to wear. Poor muscle control and difficulty with dentures can make it difficult for individuals to form words.

Aphasia, or inability to speak, is another problem affecting individuals following strokes. Left handed individuals are less likely to become aphasic as the speech centre in such individuals spans both left and right hemispheres.

Strokes can affect the vision and make reading difficult. Some individuals suffer from hemi-enopia, loss of half the vision in each eye. Sometimes words make no sense to an individual. Strokes can paralyse limbs and can cause individuals to lose the ability to write.

Individuals who are unable to communicate their needs verbally or by writing are very vulnerable. Some older people experience difficulties not only in communicating but also eating and swallowing. Such individuals can become angry and frustrated or sink into depression.

Many people can recover most if not all speech following a stroke. Recovery is dependent on the severity of the stroke, on therapy from speech therapists, on the individual's motivation and the nursing intervention.

Speech and language therapists

Speech therapists are now known as speech and language therapists (SALTS). This change of name more accurately reflects their role, which is to work with people who have problems not only with speaking but also with understanding speech and interpreting written work. The nurse can refer individuals directly to the SALT in most areas of the UK, though it is wise to check local policy. SALTS have long fought to retain a policy of open access to their services. This policy ensures that individuals, parents (in the case of children), carers and professionals can readily obtain the services of SALTS. It means that the nurse can refer either by speaking to the SALT, leaving a message on an answerphone or writing a note.

Whilst some community trusts employ SALTS, the majority are still based in hospital but cover a specific area of the community. The therapist normally makes an initial assessment visit, identifies the individual's problems, and plans care. SALTS can be asked if they wish to make notes in the individual's care plan. Most are keen to do so, and documenting the work of all professionals involved in an older person's care helps ensure continuity of care. The SALT works with the individual and the nursing staff involved in caring for the individual, to ensure that everyone is using the same methods to communicate, and working towards the same ends.

If primary nursing is used at the nursing home the primary nurse should if possible be on duty when the initial assessment takes place. The therapist may give the individual details of exercises to be carried out to improve fine muscle control to the mouth and lips; a communication card may be supplied so that the individual can point to everyday items. The nurse can begin a scrapbook which has one picture, such as a bath, on each page, with the word 'bath' written clearly and in large letters underneath. This can be used to increase the range of needs an individual can communicate.

SALTS normally decide how often they will visit after the initial assessment visit; it is usually once or twice weekly. Therapists emphasize that nursing staff have an important role to play in helping individuals with language problems to communicate, and they suggest that nurses ensure that all staff and relatives:

- speak slowly
- use simple clear language
- use short sentences
- only ask one question at a time
- only give one piece of information at a time
- use gestures
- encourage the individual to use gestures
- encourage the individual to speak
- listen and be patient

Useful address and telephone number

Local speech and language therapist

Obtaining aids

Many older people require aids to enable them to carry out the activities of daily living. A walking frame can enable an older person to walk safely around a home, and will reduce the risk of falling. Older people who are unable to grip walking frames, perhaps because of arthritis, can benefit from a gutter frame. Some older people lack the physical strength required to lift a frame and benefit from a walking frame with wheels. Individuals who have suffered from strokes and who have a residual hemiplegia, or marked weakness of one arm, are seldom able to manage a walking frame. A tripod often helps such individuals to walk.

Individuals who suffer from arthritis, or other conditions which make it difficult for them to bend, can find a Helping Hand aid invaluable. This is a long, thin, flat stainless steel aid which has two claw like pincers at the end. It can be used to pull up stockings, pick up items which are out of reach and even, with practice, change television channels.

The policy on obtaining aids varies from region to region. In some areas physiotherapists are responsible for ordering aids whilst in others this is the responsibility of the occupational therapist. It is important that individuals are assessed and the correct aid to help is selected.

People come in all shapes and sizes and it is important that the walking frame supplied is the right height for the individual. Too high a frame on a small person encourages tip toe walking and poor balance, and can lead to falls. Too small a frame for a tall person leads to the individual hunching over the frame; this leads to poor posture and the individual tends to hang their head. This often means that the individual cannot see ahead clearly and can easily fall or collide with others.

A walking frame with wheels is a boon to a weak arthritic individual but can be a hazard when supplied to an older person who tends to move fast. The individual can easily fall or collide with others.

Some tripods have the facility for the handle to be turned around so that they can be used either right or left handed; others do not. The individual who has a hemiplegia should have a tripod supplied which is of a suitable height and is designed for the appropriate hand.

The nurse should check who is responsible for supplying aids in her area and how these are obtained. In some areas the nurse may be required to fill out a form and in others she may simply telephone or write a note asking for an assessment for the individual with a view to supplying a certain aid.

It is important that older people are supplied with aids which are appropriate to their needs, but these can easily become mixed up in a home. Two individuals can sit down to lunch with their frames placed side by side; after lunch they could both pick up the wrong frame. The easiest way to ensure that individuals retain their own aids is to name each aid. This can appear very institutional so the nurse may prefer to label the underside of an aid. Some older people, though, prefer a large clearly written or printed label to be visible on their aid, enabling them to identify it readily. Some older people prefer to personalize their aids in a variety of ways; some have stickers whilst others might prefer to have a ribbon or an artificial flower tied to the aid.

Useful address and telephone number

Person and department responsible for supplying aids

Obtaining repairs

Most community health trusts have a community supplies department (known in some areas as medical loans). This is often situated at the central offices of the health trust. The community supplies department normally keeps records of the names and addresses of individuals, and details of the aids supplied to them. The rubber ends which are attached to walking frames and tripods are called ferules. These often wear down and the metal from the frame is in direct contact with the floor. Worn down ferules destabilise frames and can predispose an individual to falls. All equipment can be returned to the community supplier department for repair. Unfortunately repairs can take some time; delays normally vary from three days to three weeks and are dependent on staffing levels and current workload. Community supplies departments will make every effort to supply replacement aids if repairs cannot be carried out quickly. If ferrules are worn down the nurse can contact community supplies, give the individual's name, address and the aid. The supplies department can identify the type of aid and post ferrules to the home where these can be quickly replaced by the home's maintenance staff. It is not usually possible to remove ferrules from unused aids as there are several different sizes and fitting the wrong size can lead to accidents.

Useful address and telephone number

Community supplies department responsible for supplying and repairing aids

Wheelchairs

Some individuals bring their own wheelchairs to the home. Normally the community supplies department keeps a register of all individuals who have been issued with wheelchairs. The nurse should inform community supplies, preferably in writing and retaining a copy, of the individual's change of address. This is important as contractors asked to repair wheelchairs are supplied with a list by community supplies and will only repair chairs if details of the individual match their records. Individuals who are admitted from out of the local area must have their chairs registered with the local community supplies department for the same reason.

In most areas the individual's doctor must complete a wheelchair request form before a wheelchair is supplied. The procedure varies from area to area. In some areas this form is sent to the physiotherapist who assesses and measures the individual and orders the appropriate wheelchair. In other areas the form is sent direct to community supplies who employ contractors to assess the individual, measure them and supply the appropriate wheelchair. Your local community supplies department or physiotherapist can advise you of local procedure.

Each home is supplied with a list of individuals and the type and serial number of each wheelchair. This list should be kept in a safe place. Each wheelchair should be identified with the individual's name. Some older people may wish to use stickers to personalize their wheelchairs. This often enables them to identify them quickly.

It is important that the nurse ensures that wheelchairs are kept in a state of good repair. Flat tyres can make it difficult for individuals or nursing staff to propel the chairs. Tyres should have a reasonable amount of tread and will need replacing from time to time. Flat or badly worn tyres can affect the brakes and can mean that a chair can move despite the brakes being on. This can lead to falls and injury. Footplates should move easily and sides should slip off easily to enable older people to transfer easily. Chairs should fold without difficulty.

Ensuring that wheelchairs are well maintained makes it easier for older people who are wheelchair dependent to move freely around the home. Relatives are also more willing to take an older person on trips and outings when they are not forced to struggle with a wheelchair which is difficult to push because of flat tyres, or is difficult to fold and place in the boot of the car.

The home's maintenance staff can ensure that tyres are pumped up and that moving parts are oiled. The policy for having repairs carried out varies from area to area. In some areas community health trust staff visit the home and carry out repairs or take the chair away for major repairs or replacement. In other areas the community trust has appointed contractors to carry out such repairs. The nurse should check what the arrangements are in the local area.

When repairs are required the nurse should contact the appropriate repair staff. Details of the individual's name and the wheelchair identification code are required. If the nurse is unable to supply the serial number or identification code which has been supplied, repairs are delayed.

Useful address and telephone number

Local trust/contractor responsible for repairing wheelchairs

Exercise sessions

In many nursing homes little priority is given to providing recreational facilities for older people. Nursing staff are often so busy providing care that there is little time or thought given to social activities. But these are an extremely important part of daily life and help individuals to lead happy and fulfilled lives. Research indicates that older people who engage in activities and live life more fully enjoy better physical health. Older people who moved from NHS long stay care to an NHS nursing home benefited from the change in atmosphere and the availability of recreational activities. Many aspects of these individuals' health, including mobility and continence, improved[4].

Exercise is important at all ages and many older people benefit from regular exercise. EXTEND (Exercise Training for the Elderly and Disabled) is a registered charity which trains exercise teachers. EXTEND teachers specialize in working with older people. All older people, including those individuals who are wheelchair bound or extremely frail, can take part in EXTEND classes. Music is an important part of the classes, which have a carefully graded programme of exercises tailored to the differing abilities of individuals within the class. The programme comprises a number of exercise sequences, each one exercising a different part of the body and all designed to mobilize muscles and joints. EXTEND teachers usually work on a sessional basis and visit nursing homes once or twice per week. Nurses can obtain details about local EXTEND teachers from:

EXTEND
1a North Street
Sheringham
Norfolk NR26 8LJ.
Telephone 01263 822479.

A stamped addressed envelope is appreciated if requesting information.

Recreational activities

Recreational activities are important if the nursing home is to feel like home and not an institution. Older people who live in nursing homes come from many different backgrounds and have different interests. Recreational activities should reflect this. If possible the home should employ an activities co-ordinator to work with older people and nursing staff to organize a variety of activities. The activities co-ordinator can be a part-time appointment. If it is not possible to employ an activities co-ordinator it may be possible to find a volunteer or a number of volunteers who would be willing to co-ordinate activities within the home.

Homes who employ an activities co-ordinator should also supplement this with volunteers and members of the local community. The local citizens advice bureau (CAB) can give details of organizations who keep registers of volunteers willing to offer their time and skills. Local churches and organizations such as the Rotary Club are often keen to become involved in voluntary activities within the home.

Local clubs and societies may be willing to come to the home and give a talk or show slides. The local Society for the Protection of Birds may be able to give a talk to the elderly bird-watcher. The older person who enjoys chess but cannot find anyone in the home to play may find a partner from the local chess club who will come in and play. Volunteers come from all walks of life; newly retired people, people who are studying for professional qualifications part-time, mothers of school age children and unemployed people offer a wealth of skills.

One volunteer may be able to offer painting lessons, another flower arranging, another may be able to play the piano (if the home has one) or an electronic organ, and offer sing-songs. Volunteers can also befriend individuals who do not have a family and can visit for a chat. An older person who has a particular interest and who is visited by a member of, for example, the local amateur photographer's association may become involved in the social activities of the group. Activities and involvement with local groups can enrich an older person's life, and a life that has seemed empty and worthless can become full and enjoyable.

Many people when they consider recreational activities think of group activities. Individual activities and activities involving small groups are also important. Many older people find it difficult to take part in activities because of disabilities. It is possible to get games which have been modified to enable people with poor vision or poor muscle control to take part, for example, Scrabble is available with large tiles, and larger than normal playing cards are available.

Reading

Many older people enjoy reading. Library books and a range of daily newspapers should be available in the home. Local councils provide a special service to nursing homes. Normally the home registers with the local library service, and the librarian visits and explains about the range of books available. There are thousands of titles available in large print, and most of the books delivered can be large print. Normally the library offers a selection of books such as crime, adventure, romance, historical etc. The nurse can ask older people what type of books they like and who their favourite authors are. The library service will include these books in the selection sent to the home. Library books are normally changed every three months but the service can visit more frequently if required.

Useful address and telephone number

Local library service

Books and newspapers for the blind

Many older people who are no longer able to read can still enjoy books and newspapers. Many books are available on tape and cassette and are provided by the Talking Book Service. Individuals must be registered as blind or partially sighted to qualify for this service. The local council is required to keep a register of such individuals. Nurses who wish to obtain talking book services on behalf of individuals should contact the local council who can supply details.

A local member of the Royal National Institute for the Blind normally visits the individual and notes the reading/listening preferences; these are used to choose suitable books. Tapes are posted to the individual in a padded plastic pouch; when the tape is to be returned the label is reversed (the sender's address is printed on the back) and returned post free.

The Royal National Institute for the Blind (RNIB) can provide details of the local Talking Books group and can offer help and advice on recreational activities for blind and partially sighted individuals.

RNIB
224 Great Portland Street
London W1N 6AA.
Telephone 0171 388 1266.

Useful address and telephone number

Talking Books service

Films and television programmes

Many older people visited the cinema frequently in their youth. They often enjoy watching films from the 1920s, 1930s, 1940s and 1950s. Many films which interest older people are shown either mid afternoon or very late at night. In the afternoon the home can be busy or visitors can interrupt an enjoyable film. If the home has a video recorder, staff (and relatives) should be encouraged to find out what type of films the older people enjoy and to record these films. Video hire shops often stock older type films which can be hired inexpensively. Showing films in the evening can encourage older people to sit up, chat and enjoy an evening's entertainment.

Music

Music has a powerful effect on mood and many people enjoy listening to their favourite music. Older people can be encouraged to bring their favourite records and tapes and these can be played in the lounge, the dining area or in the individual's room. Many older people enjoy hearing music played quietly in the dining room at meal times.

Outings

Everyone enjoys going out and older people are no exception. It need not involve a great deal of planning. The nurse should encourage individuals living in the home to get out and about. The home may have a policy, perhaps because it is beside a busy road, that older people should be accompanied when they go out. Nursing staff and relatives should be encouraged to take the older person out of the home. A trip to the local coffee shop, a visit to a shop to choose toiletries, or popping into the pub for a pint, can be enjoyable trips out. Relatives would often like to have their loved one home for tea or a meal at weekends, but hesitate to suggest this to nursing staff. The nursing staff who work with relatives can suggest that the family might wish to take the individual on outings.

Local churches, charities and other organizations often arrange special trips for older people living in nursing homes. The nurse should encourage such invitations; staff, relatives and volunteers can help at such events if required.

Working with patients

Establishing regular meetings with patients enables nurses to ensure that all services within the home, including recreational services, meet the needs of individuals living in the home.

Celebrations and special occasions

It is important that individuals are able to continue celebrating special occasions such as Christmas, Easter and birthdays when they live in nursing homes. Older people and their families should be involved in planning such events. Providing a cake and cards and singing *Happy Birthday* can make an older person who entered the nursing home fearful and apprehensive, finally feel that they are 'at home' and among friends.

Conclusion

Many older people who enter nursing homes benefit from rehabilitation, which can improve quality of life. The older person and nurse can work together to determine the aims and priorities of the older person. The nurse can co-ordinate and continue the work of other professionals to enable older people to fulfil their potential. Rehabilitation and activities can transform an older person's life and enable the individual to lead a full life within the home. The nurse's role is essential to this process.

References

(1) Nazarko, L. (1993) Out of the darkness. *Elderly Care*, **5** (3) 8.
(2) Bosanquet, N. & Gray, A. (1989) *Will you still love me? New opportunities for health services and elderly people.* National Association of Health Authorities Research paper no 2. NAHA, Birmingham.
(3) Williams, E.L., Savage, S., McDonald, P. & Groom, L. Residents of private nursing homes and their care. *British Journal of General Practice*, 42, 477–81.

(4) Bond, J. (1984) An evaluation of long stay accommodation of elderly people. In *Gerontology and Social Behavioural Perspectives* (ed. D.B. Bromley). Croom Helm, London.

Chapter 13
Respite Care

Introduction

An estimated seven million people care for older people at home[1]. The majority of older people receiving care are in their 80s and 90s and are cared for by daughters, sons and other members of the family. The majority of carers are themselves in their 60s and 70s and may have health problems. Most carers provide care week after week and month after month without help or respite. Many carers have not had a night's unbroken sleep for years. Carers often find themselves unable to do things which we take for granted, such as go shopping, without a great deal of planning and organization. Carers who provide care without help eventually find that their own physical and psychological health suffers. Many older people are admitted permanently to nursing homes because the carer has become ill or can no longer continue to provide care.

The aim of respite care is to ensure that carers have a break from caring. This break may be on a regular planned basis. The older person may have two weeks respite care followed by six weeks at home. In some cases respite care is organized because the carer can no longer cope, perhaps because of illness or exhaustion. The aim of respite care is to enable an older person to return home once the crisis which made admission necessary has been resolved.

Nursing homes are now being asked to provide respite care much more than before. There are a number of reasons for this. In the past the NHS offered many carers respite facilities. NHS changes and the introduction of the internal market has led many trusts to reduce the number of respite beds within their area. Social Services Departments also offered respite beds with their part three homes. Many SSDs are now reducing the number of part three beds within their area and have few respite beds available.

The introduction of the Community Care Act led to increasing numbers of older people who would have been cared for in nursing and residential homes in the past, being discharged home. Carers are now looking after older people who are requiring greater levels of care than before. The CCA gave local authorities a responsibility to identify need within the community. The publicity which accompanied the introduction of the Act made many carers aware, for the first time, of respite services. Demand for respite care has increased over the last two years whilst respite beds in social services and NHS facilities have been reduced, so demand for nursing home respite care has increased. The provision of respite care in nursing homes is still very new although other countries such as Sweden provide almost equal numbers of long stay and respite beds. The number of respite beds in nursing homes is not known, although it seems certain that numbers will grow over the next few years as SSDs seek to contain costs, and the numbers of people surviving into extreme old age grow.

The older person's view of respite care

Older people can feel extremely anxious about the prospect of being admitted to a nursing home for respite care. The older person would usually prefer to remain at home. The prospect of entering a home rarely appeals. The home may be clean, bright and nicely decorated but the older person often feels they are being 'put away'. In an emergency situation when the carer is no longer able to cope, admission can take place within a few hours. The older person who was happy at home is suddenly told that they *have* to be looked after in a home until the situation is resolved. Many older people fear that they will never again leave the nursing home and that they have been dumped.

The nurse must be sensitive to the older person and must be aware of the fears and anxieties which often accompany such admissions. The nurse must, however, be careful not to reassure an older person that they will definitely return home if this may not be possible. The nurse should be open and honest with the older person; giving assurances about circumstances which are outside the nurse's control can be unethical and will adversely affect the nurse/patient relationship.

Planned respite care is less traumatic for the older person. The individual has an opportunity to meet the staff and patients, see the room and find out about the home before admission. The older person may still fear that respite care may become permanent; these fears are normally allayed after the first successful period of respite care.

Older people often benefit enormously from a period of respite care. Assessment by the nurse often uncovers ongoing problems or unmet needs which can begin to be met during the period of respite care. This care can be continued on discharge.

Betty McKay was admitted to a nursing home for respite care whilst her daughter attended her son's wedding in Australia. On admission Betty was wearing incontinence pads. She visited the toilet *every* 15 minutes but leaked in between. Her daughter explained that Betty hadn't had a proper night's sleep for some months because she had to keep going to the toilet. Betty's doctor had said it was due to her age and the fact that she'd had six children. A continence assessment revealed that Betty was faecally impacted and a urine specimen sent for culture and sensitivity indicated that she also had a urinary tract infection. Disimpaction, dietary advice and a diet rich in fibre ensured that Betty opened her bowels regularly and did not suffer from constipation.

Antibiotic therapy, advice about fluids, an adequate fluid intake and advice on wiping herself from front to back to avoid reinfection resolved the urinary tract infection. Betty found that she only needed to go to the toilet every couple of hours and only had to get up once in the night to pass urine. Her general health improved and she was no longer forced to rely on pads for protection. Betty enjoyed meeting people of her own age and taking part in the activities of the home. She returned home having benefited from her period of respite care.

The carer's view of respite care

Carers often only consider asking for respite care when they have reached the end of their tether. The carer is often exhausted and angry that they have been left to care alone for so long without help. At the same time the carer often feels guilty that they are no longer able to cope and they are convinced that no one will be able to provide care of the same standard as that given at home. Carers are sometimes criticized by other family members for seeking respite care.

The carer enters the nursing home with mixed emotions and can appear prickly and extremely critical. The empathic nurse will be aware of the carer's feelings and will do everything possible to allay fears, anxieties and guilt. Some carers fear that nurses will secretly condemn them for being weak and unable to cope. Nurses who recognize the carer's achievement in caring for the older person, perhaps saying, 'You've done a marvellous job but you must be looking forward to a break', can help the carer to come to terms with fears and anxieties.

Carers benefit from a break and from having time to do what they want without having to worry about caring for the older person. Carers who have access to respite care are able to continue providing care for longer. Often respite care enables the carer to continue providing care at home without ever seeking long term admission. Nurses are also aware of services which would help a carer when the older person returns home. They can help carers gain access to services or can persuade carers to accept services which have been offered but declined.

The nurse's view of respite care

Respite care is a new, challenging and rewarding development in nursing homes. In the past, many older people entered nursing homes and remained there until death. Even older people who had recovered well after illness were unable to return home because the services they required in the community did not exist.

Respite care enables nurses to assess and offer care to older people and their carers. Older people often show physical and psychological improvement when they receive skilled nursing care. Carers also benefit, changing from the terse individual who appears strained almost to breaking point, to a more contented and relaxed individual.

Nurses looking after individuals on regular respite schemes find that it takes the older person some time to settle into the home and build a relationship with staff and patients. If a few individuals are using the same respite bed on a rota basis a number of things can help each individual settle into the home more easily on admission and readmission. Carers can be asked to provide personal possessions which remain in the home. A colour photocopy (or a print if the negative is available) in a picture frame, like the one the older person has at home, a bedspread, a table lamp and other treasured items as similar as possible to the ones at home, can be supplied to the nursing home. These items can be placed in the room prior to admission so that it looks as if they have been brought from home and the room has been undisturbed since the individual's last stay. Surrounding the older person with belongings from the home environment makes the room homely and welcoming.

When the individual is returning home these items can be placed in a cardboard box with the person's name on it and stored until readmission. The room can then be repersonalised for the next readmission.

The use of primary nursing ensures that the older person is able to build up a relationship with the primary nursing team more readily than with a large group of nurses. Admissions should, whenever possible, be planned so that the primary nurse (or a member of the primary nursing team) are present. This ensures continuity of care and both older adults and their carers find this reassuring.

Respite care can make a real difference to the physical and psychological health of older people and their carers. Providing that care is incredibly rewarding and is a real morale booster for nurses.

Social services' view of respite care

Social Services Departments (SSDs) are responsible under the Community Care Act for identifying need and purchasing services to meet the identified need. They have been allocated funds from central government to enable them to purchase care.

Respite care is crucial if SSDs are to meet their responsibilities under the CCA. SSDs must develop a strategy which offers a range of care to take account of the needs and wishes of older people and their carers. Respite care allows SSDs to use resources prudently. Funds which would provide one long term care place can be used to provide four respite care places if two weeks respite is offered every eight weeks. Respite care enables carers to continue to provide care for as long as possible and can postpone or eliminate the need for long term care. Older people are able to remain where they want to be – at home – and carers who are able to have regular breaks are less likely to suffer ill health themselves.

SSDs who offer regular respite care will be informed by care managers of an individual's condition and how the family are coping. Extra services can be offered to support carers who are experiencing difficulties. Respite care can be increased, a stay of a few months organized, or permanent care planned if this is required. SSDs can plan budgets more effectively, and can plan a programme of care that will reduce the need for crisis interventions which are traumatic for older people and their carers and disrupt care managers' normal work pattern.

Problems associated with respite care

Respite care should be planned and every effort should be made to ensure continuity of care on each admission. NHS respite services ensured that the older person always returned to a designated respite bed on the same ward. SSD respite care used a similar system. Some SSDs have made every effort to ensure that older people receiving respite care in nursing homes receive such continuity of care. They have contracted with one or more homes to provide respite beds.

The SSD purchaser negotiates and agrees a price with the nursing home, who provide a respite bed for the use of the SSD. The home is paid an annual fee for the bed, which is reserved exclusively for the use of the SSD for respite care. Care managers meet their team leader and determine which of their clients require rotating respite care and the frequency of respite required.

The individuals and the carers are invited to visit the home, meet patients and staff and decide if they wish to take the place offered. A rota of three or four individuals and dates of admission and discharge is drawn up. A copy of this rota is given to the home, the individuals who are booked for respite care, and carers. Regular planned respite care in the same home ensures continuity of care and enables nurses, older people and carers to build up a relationship.

Unfortunately some SSDs have not yet contracted with homes for regular respite care and organize it on an ad hoc basis. This is time consuming as care managers can spend hours searching for a bed which is booked for a set period, usually a fortnight. There is no opportunity for nurses to build up a relationship with the individual in such circumstances. In some cases the bed is booked for another individual for a fortnight but the same individuals rarely return to the home due to poor management. This conveyor belt system of respite care is fraught with difficulty and older people can feel unhappy and unsettled by frequent changes of home. This system does not enable carers to plan a break and does little to allay their anxieties at leaving their loved one. Nurses find such respite care less rewarding than planned rotating respite care.

Sometimes rotating respite care fails to work to plan. A carer may telephone at 11 AM to say they feel unable to continue to provide care. The next planned respite admission is due at 2 PM. The carers of the individual who is due for admission have booked their first holiday abroad in five years and there are no empty beds in the home. Intervention and the offer of respite care before carers reach breaking point can help avoid such problems.

Sometimes an individual can become ill and is too unwell to be discharged or transferred. In such circumstances the care manager, team leader or duty social worker should be contacted immediately.

Contracting with social services

Some Social Services Departments advertise the fact that they wish to contract with nursing homes for respite care. Usually a set number of beds is advertised for individuals who require Elderly Mentally Infirm (EMI) and Elderly Infirm care. Homes apply for a copy of a form which is completed and the home is visited prior to contracting. SSDs who are arranging care on an ad hoc basis may welcome an approach from a home willing to contract to provide respite services. It is important to establish who will be responsible for providing transport to and from the home. It is also important to determine who will be responsible for deciding which individuals will be admitted to the home and for ensuring that the SSD provide written notice of such admissions.

If an SSD merely contracts with a home and circulates all care managers with details of the respite provision at the home, problems may arise. Each care manager may work out a rota and the number of respite places booked may far exceed the number contracted. The home may receive calls from several care managers who have all promised carers respite care over the same period. Care managers may compete with each other for places or book 26 patients into the home over a year so that each of their carers has a break. A break of two weeks a year is of little use to carers and may lead to increased demand for long term care.

The contract should include contingency plans if an individual is unable to be discharged due to illness or if the carer is unable to continue providing care. Contracts are normally placed for one year.

Supporting carers

Some carers find that their lives are empty when the older person enters the nursing home for respite care. Such carers normally visit within a few days of admission and stay for hours. They often offer to help nursing staff not only with caring for their own loved one but also with other residents. They offer to lay tables, serve meals, give out tea and help in any way possible. Some carers, especially those who have been living alone with the older person, have gradually lost touch with their friends. Leisure interests have been dropped and the carer's life has centred around the loved one. Carers can suddenly feel that their life has lost all purpose when the older person is admitted for respite care.

Planned respite care gives carers an opportunity to rebuild their lives and to expand their horizons once again. Carers may feel that they should come to the home and offer help; this situation should be handled with great care and tact. The nurse does not want the carer to feel that she is unwelcome but does not want to make the carer feel that she must visit daily and help out. In some cases the carer wants the nurse to give her 'permission' not to visit daily. The carer needs to come to terms with her wish to rebuild her own life without feeling that she has failed to care for the older person.

Most areas of the country have local carer support groups. Details are available from care managers, the local community health council or the local library. Carer support groups meet regularly and in addition to providing support also have social functions. They usually offer a 'sitter scheme' and a volunteer gets to know the older person and the carer. The volunteer arranges to come and stay at the house while the carer attends carer support meetings or goes out. Carer support groups usually have volunteer drivers who can give carers lifts to local meetings.

Many carers find that attending carer support groups helps to combat the terrible sense of isolation which can affect them. It also helps them to work through feelings of guilt and anxiety and provides a support network.

Useful name and address

Local carers' support network

Liaising with other professionals and organising services

The nurse may discover that an older person admitted for respite care has been experiencing problems which require ongoing care. The older person may be unable to get into the bath at home, even with the carer's help. The procedures for organizing assistance with bathing vary from area to area. In some areas the district nursing team are responsible for organizing baths; in other areas district nursing services only take responsibility for 'medical baths' and social services departments take responsibility for 'social baths'. 'Medical baths' are baths that are required for medical reasons, for example because an individual has a continence problem, and are provided as part of NHS care. Individuals receiving 'social baths' are charged a fee if they have savings of over £8000. Charges range from £4.50 to £6.50 nationally.

The individual may require special footwear to accommodate oedema or bunions. The individual may be deaf and require an audiology appointment. Physiotherapy may help to improve mobility or reduce pain. Speech therapy may be required to help an individual to communicate. The older person may benefit from a walking aid. Details of how to obtain these services are given in Chapter 11.

It is important when obtaining these services that the nurse writes a letter which is enclosed with the doctor's letter, giving details of the older person's whereabouts. This can state, for example:

'Mrs Daniels will be at her own home from 1st of February until 14th of March; from 14th to 28th of March she will be resident at the nursing home'.

Both addresses and contact numbers should be given. This prevents individuals missing appointments because the letter has been sent to the home address and the individual is in the nursing home while the carer has gone away. Arranging ongoing services is extremely difficult if respite care is arranged on an ad hoc basis and the individual is admitted to a number of different homes.

The older person may have enjoyed mixing with others and may confess that she sometimes feels lonely at home and will miss the company. She may benefit from attending a luncheon club, a social services day centre or a day hospital once a week. The choice available will be dependent on the individual's ability, the facilities available at each place and availability of places. Some SSD run day centres will not accept any older people who have continence problems, have difficulty in walking or who require help going to the toilet, whilst others accept individuals requiring such help. Some NHS day hospitals have strict admission criteria and will only accept individuals requiring active treatment for limited periods. Nurses should check what facilities are available locally and on the criteria for acceptance.

Arranging discharge

In a planned rotating respite scheme, discharge dates are agreed prior to admission. If the older person becomes ill and is too unwell to return home this should be discussed with the individual, the carer (if available), the doctor and the care manager. If respite was arranged for a limited period on an emergency basis, perhaps because the carer was ill, and the carer is still unwell, this should be discussed. It may be possible in these circumstances to extend the stay or to delay a planned admission.

The nurse should ensure that if the individual is taking prescribed medication, enough to last at least a week is given to the individual or the carer on discharge. If the older person has been having treatment from a district nurse the district nurse should be informed of discharge. A letter should be sent if the wound has improved or changed significantly, or if different dressings are being used. If they are, a few dressings should be supplied for the district nurse to use. The nurse should ensure that the individual's doctor is aware of the person's whereabouts; providing details of the dates of planned respite can reduce paperwork.

Conclusion

Every Social Services Department should offer respite care as part of a range of facilities which fulfil the needs and respect the wishes of older people who wish to live at home, and of carers who wish to continue providing care at home. Respite care should normally be planned and offered on a regular basis. This enables older people to live at home whilst benefiting from ongoing assessment and care from nurses. Older people and carers are often anxious when respite care is first offered. Nurses should make every effort to allay anxieties and ensure continuity of care. Working with older people, carers and other professionals to ensure that older people can continue to live at home is rewarding for the nurse.

Reference

(1) *Listening to Carers* (1992) Carers National Association, London.

Chapter 14
Palliative Care and Death

Introduction

The goal of skilled nursing care is to provide care which enhances or maintains an individual's quality of life. Reports from the Association of Directors of Social Services indicate that older people who are now being admitted to nursing homes are more acutely ill than ever before. In some areas of the country 30% of all older people admitted to nursing homes die within a month of admission. It is important that nurses are able to work with other professionals to enable older people to die without pain in a dignified way. This chapter aims to help nurses ensure that older people's spiritual needs are met and pain controlled. Details of legal requirements relating to death, and information on arranging funerals, are also given.

Pain management

Recently a colleague asked older people in the nursing home where she works if they suffered from pain. Three quarters of the individuals replied that they were frequently in pain but only 20% of these individuals told nursing staff about their pain. Most individuals who did not report pain felt that little could be done to help and there was no point in bothering the nurses.

Pain can affect every aspect of an individual's life. Individuals suffering from unrelieved pain may not wish to eat, move around or talk to others, and can become extremely depressed. Controlling pain can enhance an older person's quality of life and enable them to enjoy life once again.

Nurses cannot always rely on older people to report pain and they should observe individuals for signs of pain. Nurses should always ask if they suspect patients are in pain. The nurse is in a unique position to monitor the effectiveness of prescribed analgesia and should inform the individual's doctor if analgesia is ineffective.

Specialist pain control services

If an individual's pain cannot be controlled, specialist help should be sought. Many hospitals run pain control clinics. Individuals can visit the clinic if they are able, or a member of the community or hospital pain control team can visit the home. Pain control teams use a range of surgical and medical treatments in addition to drugs, and can normally ensure that individuals remain free of pain.

Specialist palliative care nurses normally work alongside medical staff and provide help, advice and support to individuals suffering from pain and nursing staff caring for them. In some areas palliative care nurses who work at the pain clinic work in both hospital and community settings. In other areas there are two teams, one for the hospital and another for the community. The local hospital and community health trust will be able to provide details of pain clinics and specialist palliative care nurses.

Useful addresses and telephone numbers

Pain clinic

Specialist palliative care nurse

Listening to the patient

Many older people living in nursing homes come to regard the home as 'home' and fellow patients and nursing staff as friends. Many individuals wish to die in familiar surroundings and among friends. Nurses should make every effort to ensure that the wishes of older people who wish to end their days in the nursing home are respected.

Charles Scott lived in a nursing home. One morning the nurse who was bathing him noticed that his feet were rapidly turning navy blue. Both Charles' legs were navy blue up to the knees by the time the ambulance arrived a few minutes later to take him to the local hospital. Surgeons at the hospital diagnosed a saddle embolus which was completely blocking the arteries supplying Charles' legs. The surgeons felt that Charles would not survive any attempt to remove the large embolus. Intravenous morphine administered via a syringe driver controlled pain. Charles told his primary nurse and his family that although he realised that he was dying he had no wish to die in a busy hospital ward surrounded by strangers. He asked to return home to die. The nurse specialist responsible for pain control accompanied Charles back to the nursing home and showed nursing staff how to operate the syringe driver and deal with any problems. Staff were given a number so that the nurse specialist could be contacted if problems arose. The pain control specialist visited the night staff and checked that Charles remained free of pain. Charles died three days later, in the place he had come to regard as home surrounded by family and friends. His death was peaceful, dignified and in accordance with his wishes.

Rosie Beckford was no nurse's idea of a typical old lady. She lived life to the full in a nursing home despite appalling deformities caused by osteo and rheumatoid arthritis. Rosie normally had her hair dyed bright orange but occasionally had it dyed pink, blue or mauve to match her latest outfit. Rosie always wore far too much make-up and was a noisy and exuberant person. One winter she became quieter and quieter and took to her bed. She appeared to be in great pain although she never complained. Analgesia did not appear to be effective and Rosie winced and flinched when turned. The pain control specialists visited; potent analgesia was pre- scribed; relatives, fellow patients and staff prepared themselves for Rosie's death. Rosie, though, free at last from the excruciating pain that had drained her reserves, rose from her bed like a phoenix from the ashes and enjoyed a further two years of life before dying.

Supporting the family of a dying patient

No one is ever really prepared for the death of their father, mother or close relative. Death and bereavement are things that happen to other people. The family of a person who is dying can experience a whole range of emotions:

- denial – 'Dad will be all right, he's rallied before'
- mitigation – 'well, he is 84'
- anger – 'why mum, she's really enjoying life?'
- blame – 'if my sister hadn't taken mum out in the cold'
- guilt – 'I should never have gone away on holiday'.

The nurse should be aware of these emotions and should understand the devastating effect the death of a loved one can have. The nurse should spend time with the family who may wish to talk about their feelings. The family should feel free to visit at any time and to stay for as long as they wish. Some families take turns to sit with an individual so that the individual always has a family member present during the final days of an illness. Providing tea, coffee, snacks and meals is a way of showing concern. Families may wish to contact organizations which offer support and advice after the older person has died. Some suggestions are given here.

Useful addresses and telephone numbers

Age Concern have a network of over 1000 local groups, many of which provide bereavement counselling.

Age Concern
Astral House
1268 London Road
London SW16 4ER.
Telephone: 0181 679 8000.

Age Concern
4th Floor
1 Cathedral Road
Cardiff CF1 9SD
Telephone: 01222 371 566

Age Concern
57a Fountainbridge
Edinburgh EH 9PT.
Telephone: 0131 228 5656.

Age Concern
3 Lower Crescent
Belfast BT7 1NR
Telephone: 01232 245 729.

Local Age Concern Group

Cruse offers counselling, support and advice after bereavement.

Cruse – Bereavement Care
126 Sheen Road
Richmond
Surrey TW9 1UR.
Telephone: 0181 940 4818 (general enquiries)
                   0181 332 7227 (helpline 9.30 AM–5 PM,
                   Monday to Friday)

Supporting staff

Staff who are not supported find it impossible to offer support to older people and their families. Caring for individuals who are dying can be distressing and painful for staff. Staff in nursing homes build up a close relationship with individuals whom they care for. Primary nursing tends to draw patient and nurse closer together and in homes where primary nursing is practised staff support is of prime importance. Staff can feel physically tired after providing intensive nursing to an individual who is dying. They may also feel weary and upset if relatives are finding it difficult to cope and are taking their frustrations out on nursing staff.

All staff from the most junior to the most senior require support in such circumstances. All staff can help support and comfort others after the death of a patient. Staff should be able to explore and express their feelings with others and to speak frankly about their feelings. It may be appropriate to do this on a one to one basis, in a staff meeting or informally over coffee. In some circumstances ministers of religion who visit the home can be of great help in providing staff support. Some staff may find it easier to speak to ministers rather than their colleagues.

Kate Edwards had been Mrs Ethel Barnes' primary nurse for over a year. Mrs Barnes had breast cancer with boney metastases. She was a devout catholic and visited her local church weekly until she became too unwell to leave the home. The local priest, Father Cash, visited the home weekly to give Mrs Barnes communion when she could no longer attend services. When Mrs Barnes' condition worsened she was given the 'blessing of the sick' at her request. She stated that she wanted a priest called before her death.

One day Kate, her primary nurse, entered Mrs Barnes' room to find that she had died. Kate called the priest immediately and he visited. Kate was extremely upset as Mrs Barnes' wish to have the priest with her had not been met. Father Cash was able to explain to Kate that it was felt that the spirit did not immediately leave the body on death and that she had in fact fulfilled Mrs Barnes' request.

Spiritual needs

Spirituality is an important part of many people's lives. The home should make arrangements to enable older people to have their spiritual needs fulfilled. Many homes arrange for ministers of religion to visit the home on a regular basis, usually weekly, to see individuals.

One survey carried out by a nurse working in a nursing home discovered that although older people appreciated ministers visiting the home, they would prefer to visit the church, synagogue or mosque if at all possible. Older people enjoy going to church, mixing with other members of the congregation and taking part in church activities. It is often possible to arrange for them to attend church services. Many churches have some form of transport; some even have mini-buses with ramps or tail gate lifts. In other cases church members have cars and will arrange to pick up an individual or a group of individuals and take them to church.

It is essential to check that either the home, church or individual has insurance that covers such journeys. Older people who attend church services not only benefit from going out and worshipping with others but they are often able to participate in other church activities. Invitations to activities such as coffee mornings, church bazaars, plays and other activities can enrich an older person's life. Church members often become friends and in the case of older people who have no family they can visit and act as an advocate for the individual. Church members often continue to visit the home when the older person becomes too unwell to continue to visit the church.

> Miss Lucy Tucker was a lifelong church member. She had been a music teacher, played the organ and taught the junior choir for 53 years. She became frail, weak and bedbound in her final days and told her primary nurse that her greatest regret as she approached death was that she would never again hear the junior choir sing Christmas carols.
>
> On 23rd December, the day before Miss Tucker died, the junior choir slipped into her room to sing for her, as many of their parents and grandparents had. Her primary nurse said that the look on Miss Tucker's face as the choir began to sing was the highlight of her nursing career.

Older people who live in nursing homes come from a variety of backgrounds and may be of the Jewish, Muslim, Hindu or other faith. It is important that the home can help people of all faiths to continue to practise their faith within the home and to attend their usual place of worship when possible. Ministers and members of the Jewish, Moslem, Hindi, Zoroastrian and other faiths are willing to offer assistance in enabling an older person to continue to take their place in the social and religious aspects of faith. The Jewish Passover celebrations are as important to members of the Jewish faith as Christmas is to Christians. Eid, the festival which celebrates the end of Ramadan is equally important to Muslims. Diwali, the Hindu festival of light, is of prime importance to Hindus. Many families will wish to celebrate these occasions with the older person and the nurse should offer to help, perhaps by helping the individual to get ready to go out with the family for a special meal or religious service, or preparing the older person so that family and friends can visit to celebrate this special day within the home.

Useful address and telephone number

Local ministers of religion

Death – the role of the GP in certifying death

Older people living in nursing homes are normally cared for by their own GP. In practice many older people will be cared for by one local GP or one from a GP practice. When a death occurs the doctor visits and pronounces death. If the GP is able to issue a death certificate then permission is given to remove the body to a local chapel of rest. The GP may issue the death certificate immediately or, if busy, may return later to do this.

A doctor may only issue a death certificate in certain circumstances. The doctor must have seen the individual within the last two weeks, must be satisfied about the cause of death, and the individual must not have had surgery within the last twelve months. If a locum doctor is on duty, perhaps because the doctor is having an evening off, and the GP should be able to issue a death certificate on return to duty then permission is given to remove the body to a chapel of rest. If the GP is off duty and a partner from the GP practice is on call, permission is normally given to remove the body. The death certificate will be issued by the normal GP on return to duty.

If a GP is going away for more than a few days, both the GP and the doctor who will be caring for the patients during the GP's absences should visit the home, see the patients and have a handover session. This not only ensures continuity of care but also prevents the locum being forced to refer deaths to the coroner. It avoids the risk of unnecessary post mortem examinations which can cause great distress to the older person's family.

Referring deaths to the coroner

Doctors must consult the coroner in a number of circumstances:

- if the doctor has not seen the individual in the last two weeks
- if the individual has had an operation in the last twelve months
- if the doctor does not know the cause of death
- if the death is sudden, possibly the result of an accident
- if there are any suspicious circumstances.

The coroner or the coroner's officer (normally a serving police officer who has been seconded to the coroner's office for a period of time) normally discusses the circumstances of death with the GP on the telephone. The coroner normally decides if a post mortem will be required.

Post mortem examinations

The decision to carry out a post mortem examination to determine the cause of death rests with the coroner not the individual's doctor. The coroner will take into account the circumstances of death, the doctor's opinion and the wishes of the family wherever possible.

In a case where the GP has not seen the individual for more than two weeks but the individual has a long standing illness (such as terminal cancer or a heart condition) which the GP feels has caused death, the coroner may decide that a post mortem is not required.

In a case where the individual has had surgery in the last twelve months but the GP is satisfied that the operation did not directly lead to death, the coroner may decide that a post mortem is not required.

In a case where an older person has suddenly died and the GP is not able to ascertain the cause of death a post mortem *is* required. In a case where death has followed an accident or there are suspicious circumstance a post mortem *is* required.

Removal of the body

If a post mortem is required the body is not normally touched until the coroner has given permission. The coroner and/or the coroner's officer may wish to visit the home to see the body, perhaps take photographs or talk to nursing staff . The coroner normally only visits if the death may have occurred as a result of an accident or in suspicious circumstances.

When a post mortem examination is required the body is washed and dressed in a nightgown or pyjamas. Catheters, colostomy bags, dressings etc. are left untouched and the orifices are not normally packed. The nurse should consult the local coroner and check procedure in the local area. This procedure may change when one coroner leaves and another takes up post.

The body is removed by undertakers nominated by the coroner, at the coroner's expense, to the coroner's office to await post mortem. Post mortem is normally carried out within two or three working days of death. The home and family are normally notified of the result by telephone. In most cases a death certificate is issued by the coroner, the body is transferred to the firm of undertakers dealing with the arrangements, and the family can arrange burial or cremation.

Coroner's informal enquiries and inquests

In some cases the coroner may wish to ask the nursing staff a few questions relating to the circumstances of an individual's death. Many nurses become very worried and upset by the thought of being questioned informally by a coroner. The coroner is merely trying to find out about the circumstances relating to the death and is not blaming the nurse in any way. Nurses, though, often prefer to have a member of their professional organization or a friend present in such circumstances and this is perfectly reasonable.

> Mr George Blackstone had lived in a nursing home for some years. After lunch each day he walked back to his room accompanied by a nurse. One day Mr Blackstone fell backwards, struck his head on a radiator and was dead when the nurse bent down. The coroner visited the home and photographs were taken before Mr Blackstone could be moved. The coroner spoke to the nurse, Paul Henry, (in the presence of Mr Henry's professional representative) asking if Mr Blackstone had complained of being unwell before falling or if the nurse had noticed any difference in Mr Blackstone's condition that day.
>
> A post mortem revealed that Mr Blackstone had suffered a massive heart attack and had been dead before he struck his head on the radiator.

Inquests are normally to establish the circumstances, actions or inactions which led to an older person's death. Inquests take place in the Coroner's court. Nurses asked to attend an inquest should consult their professional body for further advice and support.

Last offices

The home should have a policy for last offices, which respects the individual's faith. People of the Muslim faith are not normally touched by nonMuslims after death and last offices are carried out by a person from the local mosque.

For other individual's the eyes should be closed, dentures placed in mouth and a pillow placed under the jaw for support. The body is normally left for an hour before last offices are performed. The supporting pillow is removed from the jaw.

Dressings are normally removed and wounds covered with gauze and an opaque occlusive dressing material to prevent leakage. Any catheters, drains or tubes are removed and dressings applied if required to contain leakage. The rectum may require packing with cotton wool if leakage is occurring. The body is normally washed by two members of the nursing staff, then dressed in clean night clothing, the hair is combed, and the bed remade with clean linen. Nursing staff may wish to read a prayer or poem or merely say goodbye at this stage. Members of the family may wish to see the body at this stage and say their last goodbye. The nurse must judge whether it is appropriate to remain with the family or to leave them alone. The body is then removed to a chapel of rest by undertakers until burial or cremation is arranged.

Cremations

Usually people wish to be buried or cremated locally. In some cases an individual indicates a wish to be cremated some distance from the home.

When an individual is to be cremated two doctors must examine the body of the deceased and complete a cremation form before cremation can take place. The GP usually carries out an examination, completes the first part of the form and arranges for a colleague to visit the local chapel of rest to carry out an examination and complete the second part of the form. If arrangements have been made to carry out a cremation some distance away from the home, the cremation form must be completed by *both* doctors before the body can be transported some distance. Arrangements can usually be made either for both doctors to complete their examination and fill in the cremation form before the body is transported, or for the body to remain in a local chapel of rest until these formalities have been completed.

Funerals

Many older people have come to terms with their own mortality and made arrangements for their own funeral. A widow may wish to be buried in the family plot with her husband or to have her ashes scattered in the garden of remembrance as her husband's were. Another individual may wish to be buried in the family plot. Many older people have nominated undertakers, made arrangements for and paid for their funerals. Older people who have families normally involve or inform the family of their plans. The nurse should enquire about the individual's wishes sensitively and with great tact. Any funeral arrangements should be recorded in the individual's records so that all staff are aware of them.

Some older people have no relatives and wish to make arrangements for their own funeral. They often ask the nurse for advice about organizing and paying for a funeral from their savings. The nurse should ask the older person if they wish to be buried or cremated and can then ask a number of funeral directors to provide quotations for a prepaid funeral.

There is an enormous variation in the cost of a funeral. A simple cremation can cost between £650 and £1,400 from different funeral directors within the same area. If an older person wishes to be buried in a family plot the undertaker's quotation will include the costs of re-opening the grave, placing an additional inscription on the head stone and replacing the headstone. In some cases a family plot has no further space for burial and the older person may wish to have their ashes scattered over the family plot.

If an older person wishes to be buried in a cemetery they must purchase a plot. Cemeteries are either owned by churches or local authorities or are privately owned. Charges for plots vary and cemeteries will provide brochures giving details of these.

Prepaid funerals

Many older people wish to pay for their funerals from their savings. A number of schemes exist which enable an older person or their family to make such arrangements.

Chosen Heritage Ltd is run by the trading company of Age Concern and all profits are donated to Age Concern. Three funeral plans are offered and a local undertaker is nominated to carry out the arrangements.

> Chosen Heritage
> Freepost
> East Grinstead
> East Sussex RH19 1ZA.
> Freephone: 0800 525555.

Dignity Ltd is run by Help the Aged and the Plantsbrook Group. There are four plans on offer and payment can be made by instalments if desired.

> Dignity Ltd
> Freepost
> BM2415
> Sutton Coldfield
> West Midlands BR72 1BR.
> Freephone: 0800 269318.

Golden Charter offer four plans on behalf of the Society of Allied and Independent Funeral Directors. Payment can be made by instalments.

> Golden Charter Ltd
> Crowndale House
> 1 Ferdinand Place
> Camden
> London NW1 8EE.
> Freephone: 0800 833800.

Co-operative Funeral Services offer four prepayment plans. Payments can be made by instalments.

Funeral Bond Office
Co-operative Funeral Services
Freepost
London SE18 5BR.
Freephone: 0800 289 120.

Financial help with funeral costs

Some older people and their families do not have sufficient money to pay for a funeral. In some circumstances the family of an older person may be able to get help from the Department of Social Security's social fund to help with the costs. The person applying for this grant must fulfil certain criteria.

The person taking responsibility for the funeral (*not the older person who has died*) must be in receipt of income support, family credit, disability working allowance, housing benefit or council tax benefit, or be the partner of someone receiving these benefits. Assets of the deceased are taken into account, together with any savings over £1000 of the person making the arrangements. If, for example, the funeral costs £1000 but the relative has savings of £1500, the relative will be expected to contribute £500 towards the funeral costs.

If the older person has no savings and no family, the home will be unable to claim the costs of a funeral from the DSS social fund. When a patient who has no family dies, the nurse should take legal advice regarding possessions.

Funeral arrangements for individuals who have no assets and no family

Local authorities have a legal duty under the Public Health (Control of Diseases) Act 1984 (section 46) to arrange the burial or cremation of any person who has died in their area with no assets and no family. A simple burial or cremation is arranged and a minister of religion is present. The local authority normally has an agreement with a local undertaker who organizes the funeral. These funerals usually take place early in the morning but the nominated undertaker will normally change the time if nursing staff wish to attend to pay their last respects.

When an individual dies in such circumstances the nurse should contact the local authority who will give details of the nominated undertaker and ask the home to liaise with the undertaker. Often such events occur during holidays or at weekends and it can be difficult to contact the local authority. It is sensible to inform the local authority in advance of any individuals in the home without savings, family or friends, and to obtain and keep details of the nominated undertaker.

It may not always be possible to inform the local authority in advance about individuals without savings as many older people do not wish to discuss their financial affairs with nursing staff. In such circumstances, if it is not possible to inform the local authority, the nurse can contact the nominated undertaker direct. The body can be taken to the chapel of rest and the local authority contacted when their offices are open.

When an individual without savings or family dies in hospital the health authority has a duty (HSG(92)8) to arrange and meet the cost of the funeral.

Useful address and telephone number

Local undertaker nominated by local authority

Legal formalities

When a death certificate has been issued the death must be registered. This is normally within five days of death. A member of the family usually registers the death. If the individual has no family or close friends the nurse may have to register the death.

The death should be registered in the area where the person has died and not the area where the family live or where the older person lived prior to admission to the nursing home. The death certificate and the individual's medical card are given to the registrar of births, deaths and marriages. The registrar will ask for certain information which will be included in the register of births and deaths: the full name, place and date of birth, occupation, maiden name and husband's occupation (in the case of a married woman).

The Department of Social Security produce a useful leaflet, *What to do after death* (leaflet no D49).This contains detailed information and advice and nurses may wish to give a copy to families and friends who are arranging funerals and dealing with the affairs of someone who has died. The leaflet can be obtained free from local benefit offices. Bulk copies can be obtained from:

BA Storage and Distribution Centre
Manchester Road
Heywood
Lancashire
OL10 2PZ.

Remember to quote the reference number and state the number of copies required.

The home must keep a register of deaths. Registration and inspection officers routinely ask how many deaths have occurred since the date of the last annual inspection. Although details of deaths are normally kept in the admission and discharge register, many homes also keep a separate book which states the individual's name and date of death.

Each home must provide registration and inspection officers with details of individuals who have died. Many health authorities produce a standard form and it is the duty of the nurse in charge of the shift to complete this form and post it to the local registration officers.

Discussing a resident's illness and death with other residents

Older people form deep friendships with other residents in the home. When an individual becomes ill other residents often ask how the person is. The nurse should inform the person who is ill (or the family if the individual is unable to speak) that other residents are enquiring about them, and should obtain permission to inform other residents about the individual's condition without breaching confidentiality. Some residents may wish to visit, and if the individual welcomes these visits the nurse should help residents to the room and leave them to speak privately or simply sit with the individual.

When an individual dies it is important that other residents do not see the body leave the home, as this can be distressing. Residents should be informed that the individual has died. Some may wish to attend the funeral. The nurse should work with the family and friends of those who wish to attend the funeral and should make arrangements for residents to pay their last respects.

Conclusion

The nurse's role in supporting older people and their families and ensuring that an older person's last days are without pain, is of vital importance. Sensitive care attuned to the needs of the individual enables older people to experience a dignified death and to have their needs met.

The nurse's role in helping older people and their families prepare for and come to terms with death is a demanding one. It is important that death, one of the last great taboos, is acknowledged and that residents who wish to discuss the deceased person's life are not discouraged from doing so. Residents may wish to pay their last respects and the nurse should work with relatives to enable them to do so. Nurses are only human and need to support each other and talk openly about their feelings after the death of an older person they have cared for.

Useful address and telephone number

Local coroner

Chapter 15
The Way Forward

What does the future hold for nursing homes?

It is impossible to predict the future. It is only possible to consider some ways in which nursing home care may develop.

Possible political and legislative changes

It is doubtful if any government will seek to reverse the move from NHS care to nursing home care. The demographic changes and cost involved would make any such changes extremely difficult. The experimental nursing homes set up in the early 1980s proved that nursing homes provide a humane, cost effective alternative to NHS long stay units.

The legislation concerning nursing homes will undoubtedly change within the next few years. The Registered Homes Act 1984 is vague and open to widespread local interpretation. Any future legislation would concern itself with specifying standards and ensuring nationwide uniformity. This, of course, will have cost implications and those costs will ultimately be borne by government as 60% of nursing home care is state funded. A future government may be influenced by cost implications and this may have an impact on future legislation.

The Royal College of Nursing and the British Association of Social Workers have both called for an end to the differentiation between nursing homes and residential homes. The concept of the 'single care home' is currently popular. A single care home which provides staffing levels and facilities similar to that of a nursing home would raise the costs of care significantly. It might also lead older people who do not require high levels of nursing care on admission to become institutionalized and enter the continuum which leads to excessive dependency. Nursing skills of the highest standard would be required to ensure that this did not occur.

Providing nursing home care for an additional 350 000 people (those currently cared for in residential and local authority homes) would be costly. Any such legislation would have to be phased in so that sufficient nursing staff could be trained or recruited. A single care home policy in which nurses merely supervized care assistants would deprive extremely vulnerable older people, currently cared for in nursing homes, of the benefits of nursing care. Such a proposal might well meet opposition from the public, who hold nurses and nursing in high regard and might be fearful of the consequences of unskilled people caring for the elderly.

Possible changes in nursing home inspection

There are currently two inspectorates. Residential homes are inspected by Social Services Department staff who may have a social work qualification. Nursing homes are inspected by professional nurses. There has been much debate in recent years about the wisdom (and the expense) of maintaining two separate inspectorates. It has been suggested that both inspection teams be merged.

Any such merger would be linked to legislation relating to nursing home registration and the single care home concept. It would dilute nursing skills within the nursing homes inspectorate. Many skilled professional nurses working in nursing homes would object to nursing care being evaluated by non nurses and would argue that only nurses are qualified to examine and comment on nursing care. Nursing home inspectors must demonstrate their worth at every possible opportunity if such changes are to be avoided.

The growth of large homes

Until fairly recently nursing homes were small units, but the number of beds in each has been rising. Many nursing home inspectors (and their employing health authority) sought to limit the number of beds a nursing home could provide. They argued that if nursing homes became too large they began to resemble the large geriatric hospitals they had replaced. There was a greater danger of institutionalization in larger units, which could be more impersonal than small units.

Now, corporate nursing home groups are increasingly opening large units; some have as many as 150 beds. As the size of home increases the salaries on offer to matrons increases. Until now the salaries on offer attracted nurses, and nursing homes have developed as nurse-led units. There is a danger that doctors and professional managers will be attracted by the greater salaries on offer in large nursing homes, and the nurse's role as the person in charge of nursing homes could disappear.

It is essential that nurses prove the worth not only of skilled nursing care but also the value of experienced nurse managers within a nursing home setting. Nurse managers within the NHS have failed to do this in many areas and have been supplanted by professional managers from business and retail backgrounds. We must learn from their experience if nursing homes are to remain nurse-led.

Possible changes in medical care provided to nursing home patients

The speciality of geriatric medicine was pioneered by Dr Marjorie Warren in the 1930s. It was recognized that older people could benefit from rehabilitation and active treatment rather than merely custodial care. The closure of NHS elderly care units and the increasing tendency towards integration of medical and geriatric specialities has not resulted in a reduction in the number of geriatricians employed by the NHS. Yet the majority of the most frail and disabled older people are now cared for in nursing homes.

Medical care is provided by GPs, the majority of whom do not have any specialist training in elderly care. This lack of specialist training could lead to older people within nursing homes failing to receive medical care for treatable illness. The lack of specific care by appropriately trained doctors is precisely the situation that existed when Dr Warren began her pioneering work in the 1930s. She found then that this led to unnecessary institutionalizing of older people who could be discharged home when treated and rehabilitated.

It may be that in the future, the government, alarmed by the escalating costs of institutionalizing greater numbers of older people, will investigate the reasons and at that point geriatricians will have a role in providing medical care to older people living in nursing homes. Until then, care will continue to be provided by GPs, many of whom, according to a recent survey, found their nursing home caseload 'unmanageable'.

Possible changes in the education of nursing home staff

The role of nursing homes is changing rapidly. Nurses are required to have the skills necessary to provide care to older people who are acutely ill or terminally ill, or requiring respite care, rehabilitation or long term care. The need to provide education tailored to help nurses develop and extend these skills, will be recognized. The publication of the RCN document on the qualifications and experience required by nursing home matrons is an indication that this process has begun. Eventually national Board courses linked to universities which are CATS rated, will develop.

As nursing becomes more academically focused diploma and degree courses and modules will become available. Their development may be opposed by some who feel that these needs can be met by courses designed for NHS nurses. However, as colleges of nursing seek to find business within the market-led NHS, the lure of a potential market of 70 000 nurses will lead to these courses becoming available. This may in turn lead to the development of masters degrees in nursing home care, and the emergence of the 'teaching nursing home' run by a nurse practitioner who at that point will be able to prescribe drugs and initiate nursing care and routine investigations currently the preserve of doctors.

The teaching nursing home will not only concern itself with the teaching of student nurses but also with doctors. Already Project 2000 nurses are working in nursing homes as part of their clinical placement in elderly care. Nursing homes are already beginning to forge links with colleges of education and universities. Elderly care nursing is nursing in its purest form.

The nursing home of the future primarily staffed by skilled professional nurses will be a place where nursing research is carried out, where care is developed from a holistic perspective, and where nursing models can be tried and tested. The nurse is in a unique position to work with older people, their families and other professionals to provide nursing care in centres of excellence.

Possible role of staff with National Vocational Qualifications

The introduction of Project 2000 resulted in student nurses, who had provided a great deal of care under the direction of professional nurses, no longer being part of the NHS workforce. That contribution is now limited to 1000 hours over their training period. The concept of the support worker with National Vocational Training Qualifications (NVQs), was introduced.

NVQ practical skills at level three closely mirror traditional nurse training, although trainees lack the knowledge base of registered nurses. It is possible that if nursing becomes an all graduate profession and becomes more highly paid as a result, nurses will cease to nurse. They may become supervisors and co-ordinators of care, which is delivered by staff with NVQ qualifications. This is a particular danger if nurses extend their role and at the same time divest themselves of what they perceive to be mundane and routine tasks.

It must be remembered that the extension of a nurse's role is often a result of doctors divesting themselves of what they perceive to be mundane and routine tasks. If nurses no longer nurse, care will become fragmented and it will be impossible to provide the holistic care for which every nurse should aim. In order to avoid this, nurses within the whole profession must examine the purpose and role of nursing. The profession must ensure that everyone in the country is aware that the role of the nurse is to nurse.

The future of nursing within nursing homes and within the country is uncertain. What is certain, though, is that care within nursing homes is set to change as the population ages. Nurses and nursing practice must change to meet those needs.

Index